ARE YOU READY? YOU'LL BE A DAD!

THE NEW DAD'S GUIDE TO PREGNANCY, EVERYTHING A NEW DAD NEEDS TO KNOW ABOUT HIS BABY AND MOM.

Table of Contents

Introduction *7*

Chapter 1. Support Your Pregnant Woman *9*

Getting Prepared 9
Finances 9

Helping Her Eat for Two 25
Foods She Shouldn't Eat 28

Activities to Avoid 29

Chapter 2. Importance Of The Role Of Becoming A Dad *31*

The Importance 31
What to Expect 33
How to Help 34
Identifying Feelings 36
Sex during Pregnancy 37
Overcoming Intimacy Issues 39
A Dad's Role during Delivery 40
Early Labor 40
Active Labor 40
Delivery 41

A Dad's Role after Delivery 42

Chapter 3. Home Preparations *45*

Getting the Right Gear 46
The Overwhelming World of Baby Clothes 47

Types of Baby Clothes 48
Listing the Clothes Your Baby Needs 49
Tips for Selecting Baby Clothes 52
Filling the Toy Box 54
Stroller Shopping 57
Choosing the Right Car Seat 58
Feeding, Bathing, and Entertaining 59

Making Room for the Baby 61
Finding Functional Furniture and Gear 62
Decorating the Nursery 64

Chapter 4. What A New Dad Needs To Know   67

Your Emotional Well-being in a Post-Pregnancy World.. 67

Emotions You Can Expect to Feel 68
Excitement—but Also Helplessness 68
Joy—but Also Guilt.. 69
An Outpouring of Childhood Emotions 71
A Deeper Connection to Your Partner—but Also Emotional Distance 73

Paternal Postpartum Depression.............. 74
Why It Happens 77
How to Deal With It 78

Your Relationship After Baby's Arrival 80
Common Relationship Issues 80
How to Handle These Problems 82
How to Strengthen Your Relationship After the Baby 83

Chapter 5. The Attention Of Dads For The First Time 86

Cuddle Your Baby as Often as Possible 86

Get in as Much Skin Contact as Possible... 87

Become Baby's Comforter of Second Resort 87

Make the Baby Laugh 88

Unlock Your Inner Child With the Baby 88

Talk to the Baby 89

Sing 89

Read the Baby a Bedtime Story 90

Watch Your Baby Sleeping 90

Wear the Baby 90

Take Pictures and Family Videos! 91

Fill your Role With Grace 91

Bath Time Bonding 92

Dance Together 92

Try a Baby Massage 92

Love on Your Partner in Front of the Baby 93

Take Part in Bedtime Routines 93

Practice Patience 94

Chapter 6. How To Be An Excellent Parent And Partner 95

Caring for Baby and Helping Your Partner 95

Baby Blues or Something More Serious? .. 97
    Recognize the Signs of PPD 98
    Getting Help 99

Keep Communicating! 101

How to Support the New Mom: The First Day Home 101

More Feel-Good Things Dad Can Do For Mom 103

Things Dads Do With the Baby 105

Additional Tips for Dad 106

Chapter 7. The Step By Step Guide From The Temperature Of The Bottle To The Bond With Your New Baby 112

How to Hold the Baby the Right Way 113

Popular Holding Positions: 114

How to Change the Baby 115

Bonding with the Baby 117

Skin-to-Skin Contact 117

Sing to Your Baby 118

Bathe Your Baby 118

Wear Your Baby 119

Swaddling 101 119

The Struggle of Feeding 121

Co-Sleeping 125

Crib vs. Bassinet 128

Sleeping Parents 129

Bathing the Baby 131

Don't Forget about the Pictures! 133

Chapter 8. Plan And Refine Your Childcare Style   134

> Ask For Guidance 135
>
> Get Help 135
>
> Choose A (Authoritative) Parenting Style And Stick To It 135
>
> Defend Your Personality Style................ 136
>
> Types of Dad 136

Conclusion... 143

Introduction

In today's society, men are taking more active roles in shaping the lives of their kids, as they should. Gone are the days of outdated notions about the roles of men and women in the household. Women aren't just expected to stay at home and take care of the family while men go out and look for work. These days, the delineations between the father and mother in regard to family planning and management are more blurred, and that's a good thing. It means that mothers are now free to pursue careers for themselves while dads are also free to be more immersed in their home life.

The fact that you're reading a book like this is proof that you are someone who is invested in shaping your family the right way. You aren't content with being the kind of dad who just goes to work and brings home the bacon. You want to be so much more than that, and that's amazing. Just for having that kind of mindset, you've already proven yourself to be an upstanding human being. It shows that you've got good intentions and a willingness to learn. Unfortunately, as they say about any endeavor, good intentions are not enough.

Fatherhood is the ultimate challenge, but it's also an incredible privilege that not all men are lucky enough to have. If you're expecting to bring a little child into your life soon, then congratulations. You have been blessed with the beautiful responsibility of shaping another person's life. However, that responsibility is not one you should take lightly. There's a lot that you need to learn and catch yourself up on. Fortunately, this book can serve as the perfect resource for that. Ultimately, this book is designed to get you from knowing absolutely nothing about parenting to, at the very least, gaining even just a smidge of confidence about your skills as a father.

Chapter 1. Support Your Pregnant Woman

Getting Prepared

In this chapter, we'll explore some of the things I didn't pay enough attention to the first time around. And how I wish I had! It would have saved so much hassle when we could at least deal with it - and the shock of the financial costs! I was so unprepared! So let's look at the finances first of all - hope for the best but prepare for the worst!

Finances

According to the USDA, for a middle-income family, a child costs around $13,000 every year (excluding birth costs). So if you start to budget now and prepare for this, it will come as less of a shock!

The hospital costs and medical insurance depends so much upon where you live. So first, you need to make sure what your position is. Do you need to finance a large part of the medical costs - or is it free? Will maternity leave impact the money available?

Whatever this cost comes to, there are other financial obligations, so let's go ahead and see what they are.

Life insurance

You might not want to consider what will happen to your family if you die. But, for your own peace of mind - and for your wife's - get insured. How will you manage if it is your wife who dies? Hard though these questions are, you are the man, and you have to face them. So, get the advice you need to safeguard your future and that of your unborn child. Life insurance for both you and your wife will help if the unimaginable happens.

The other costs are more exciting!

Stroller

You want to be the proud dad as you walk your newborn baby. People love babies, so don't be surprised if your grumpy neighbor crosses the road to coo at your little darling! Although you will want a nice looking stroller, the safety and functionality of the stroller is much more important. People will generally be looking at your baby instead of the stroller anyways. But the stroller needs to be sturdy and tough.

Expect to pay between $100 to $1000 for a fancy one.

One little tip - babies are interested in faces very early on. If you can safely prop up a non-breakable mirror or a picture of a face where your baby can see it, it will entertain your baby on occasion.

Keep this stroller for next time around, and invest in an umbrella-style stroller once your baby can sit up independently. (Cost $25 - $100.) Your wife will find this easier to push around, and you can lift it into the car. It is likely to get a bit worn – mud on the wheels, a drooling baby, and so on. Make sure it comes with an attachable bag for nappies and all the sundry items a baby needs. It's best if it is detachable – our first cheap stroller looked lovely in the store – but the first time we loaded it up with baby and bag, we nearly tipped the baby out, and the bag went flying when we came to unload it.

Car seat

Don't buy this second-hand – you don't know where it's been and what stresses it might have endured. Look for the safety label on your purchase. Buy it new, but you don't have to fork out for the most expensive model available. After all, your child might be car sick. Look to pay between $40 -$400. Car seats for children have expiry dates - be careful to check this out.

Baby monitor

You may think you won't need one – but it's a great standby for those moments when you and your wife are wanting a little time together. A basic model can cost as little as $20, but if you want an all-singing all-dancing model, pay up to $400. Most of us do not need this, but you might like to keep an eye on things, not only to ensure you hired the correct person to watch your little one, but you also enable you to see them when you miss them.Baby sitters

I had trouble persuading my wife to come out with me – but I was desperate to take her out to dine her and even wine her once the baby was safely delivered. I wanted to celebrate – my wife needed to know that our child was OK – all the time. (And so did I.)

After much haggling between us, we decided that we would pay top rates, check references, and come home early. We needn't have worried - a smiling face greeted us when we arrived home; our precious baby was sleeping blissfully.

Once we had found the ideal babysitter, we both agreed that paying good rates, leaving her a nice snack, and treating her with respect was worthwhile. We got to know her, and we got to trust her. She became our baby's first friend.

Diapers

Have you any idea how much diapers cost?

Disposable diapers are a boon for busy mums – total cost for a year – about $3,000.

Washable diapers – cost between $500 - $900 a year – plus extra electricity and water charges.

My clever wife made a bargain with me – "I'll wash the nappies," she said, "but you must buy me a new outfit." It seemed like a good bargain – so we had a nappy bucket nesting in the bathtub for a couple of years – and my wife looked gorgeous, and we felt we were single-handedly saving the environment.

Helpful tip from my wife: always presoak the diapers. They come out sparkling. If your state permits you to hang them outside to dry, then the extra fresh air not only makes them smell nice, but sunshine is a natural bleach and not using the dryer will save you some money on electricity.

Bassinet

Where will your little one sleep – where is the safest place. Ideally, she should be in the same room as you to sleep at least for the first six months, and a bassinet or sleeping crib gives her her own sleeping space. Research has shown that having your child sleep in your room (but not in your bed) can reduce the chance of SIDS by up to 50'%. Expect to pay anywhere between $100 - $1000.

Baby mat

Where do you put the baby when your arms are aching, or it's time to eat? Answer – on the baby mat or cushion. They need opportunities to feel the firmness of the ground, to learn to lift their head, to roll over, and so much more. A little later, you might choose to buy a baby swing – and a baby carrier or sling frees your hands as you walk around with her, as well as giving essential close contact between you and your baby. Look to be paying between $20 - $150 for these items.

One of our best buys was a baby door jumper. Of course, your baby needs to be old enough to enjoy this - usually between 6-24 months. I used to hang her on the door and watch her strengthen her little legs as she bounced around - it kept both of us amused, but never for too long (generally 10-15 minutes per day) as prolonged time can cause developmental problems in their lower body.

Formula feeds/ bottles

Your baby needs feeding! Breasts might be best - but other options should be available. You might want to try YOUR hand at feeding your infant – and you need the right equipment.

Costs here vary enormously. From nursing bras ($15 - $60) to a year's supply of formula feeding ($1200(plus accessories like bottles). Our second child had to be fed this way – and finding a bottle shape she liked was frustrating and unexpected. We went through eight different models – at an average of $8 each – and then we needed to buy eight of the chosen model – the costs can mount up.

There is nothing like feeding your baby to create a strong bond. Maybe your wife needs a rest(in fact, being well rested will help her milk supply)

- so why not let her store some of her breast milk at a convenient time for her - but you feed the baby? It gives her a break and helps you get to know your child, a win, win, win situation!

When your baby starts on solids, you will probably buy at least some jars of baby food or other foods, depending on how you plan to wean your child. A monthly extra on your grocery bill of around $50 should cover this.

Now we come to the fun stuff – the nursery, the clothes, the entertainment.

Nursery equipment /decoration/ shelves and cupboards

This is where super-dad can shine! Are you going to surprise our wife – or are you going to make it a joint venture. During this stage of her pregnancy, your wife is usually full of energy – so my advice to you dads – take advantage of it!

Once your baby outgrows the bassinet, he will need a crib. This is better bought new. There are up-to-date safety features – like the width of the bars so your baby can't trap his head, the material the mattress is made from – plus who wants to sleep in a bed where the previous occupant has peed, cried and worse?

You might be able to defer this cost – but expect to pay at least $150 and probably considerably more.

Birthdays, holidays, Christmas

We love to celebrate – any excuse. Somehow it doesn't matter if little Johnnie is too young to understand the concept of Christmas. Having children is what makes these festivals come to life.

Too many of us get a cold shower in January when we see our credit card statements. Yet this is the time to spend on next Christmas since many of the stores are trying to off-load their stocks of crackers, Santa hats, and plastic reindeer.

Plan in advance. Buy small gifts every month and put them aside for birthdays and any other celebrations. Then, you can feel smug when you see the crowds buying last-minute gifts – and you have most of yours already – and the cost is spread. I won't even attempt to put a price on this!

Fun activities

This means many things - you might think of yourself as a permanent chauffeur to football, dance classes, judo, etc., etc. but for now, just think about taking your wife out for a romantic evening. Only you know the financial standing and how much you can afford. This doesn't need to be something that is expensive, a nice walk by the river can be just as meaningful as a fancy meal and a movie. It's not the money you spend – it really is the thought that counts.

Clothes for the wife and clothes for the baby

Your wife is starting to show, to change her shape, and the baby bump is arriving. She needs some new clothes! Even more, she needs to be reassured that she is amazingly attractive.

As for your little one – vanity has yet to come. Ensure you can manage the fastenings and that they are in the right place for diaper changing. Babies like bright colors. Don't buy too many sleepers in the first size – they grow out of them. Be prepared to cut the feet, so their little toes are not squashed. Tough, cheerful, and practical is what you are looking for.

And - finally - is your home big enough?

This may not be the time to consider moving house – but sometimes you find that your home isn't big enough for three. Of course, this is a significant extra cost – but if you have to move, do it now before your baby bump gets any bigger! Or hold off for a year or so.

Now for the good news

Family, friends, and neighbors often stock unwanted toys and activity centers, just waiting for a good home. Also, garage sales may have just the perfect items, and if you plan ahead, you can take advantage of shop sales.

The first year I bought Christmas decorations at a cut-price in January, my wife thought I was crazy – but come November, and she was impressed. You might find incredible giveaways as well as useful tips to help save money at expectant parent expos - it might be worth having a look.

I think of the 7 Cs to help me remember what my wife needs in this highly emotional time for her. We needed to make a "birth plan" together.

The 7 Cs for the birth plan

- Classes

- Concerns
- Care
- Communication
- Consider
- Cesarean Section?
- Culture

Let's look at classes first

Having sorted out the monetary costs of having a baby, we can turn to the matter of prenatal classes – for you as well as your wife. She needs your support – and you need to be educated! The first time around for me, I thought – "This is women's work – I'd rather not know." I felt I would be embarrassed with all those pregnant ladies. I felt superfluous. Believe me, that was nothing compared to how useless I felt when my wife did go into labor. I was left foolishly holding her hand, grimacing when she moaned and simply getting in the way of the midwives.

How wrong I was not to go to the ante-natal classes with my partner. The second time around, I went – and I was embarrassed by how little help I had been to my adorable wife.

I learned how to help her cope with the pain. I learned how to use relaxing techniques to soothe her – pain is always worse when you are tense and anxious. I was able to help her find more comfortable positions while she was in labor. Perhaps the most helpful thing was breathing. This can be a wonderful relaxer when you know how to breathe properly – and is also an essential part of the actual birth. I never realized breathing could be so hard to do it right and how helpful it can be for the laboring woman to have someone by her side, breathing with her (it calmed me down as well). Do you know how to breathe?

As well as relaxing and breathing, I learned other things I would never have thought about. How skin-to-skin contact between mother and baby is important. (It's nice for dad, too.) I learned about how to care for my baby – but also what my partner needed to recover from the arduous work involved in the delivery of a real live baby.

The midwife teaching the class told us about how the fetus was developing, and the baby bump grew bigger. We learned about feeding options and safety – that part got me checking over my house as soon as we got home and buying safety plugs for all the sockets.

We also learned how to put a baby down to sleep. You don't just dump her in her bassinet or cot and hope she'll go to sleep quickly - you must always lie the baby down on his or her back; not on her side, not on his tummy - on their back. This reduces the risk of that terrible cot death syndrome. When I heard that, I felt truly awful - I'd usually put my precious baby down on her tummy - I could have killed her!

She also made me realize I could have saved a bunch of money if I had known then what I know now. We discussed cultural issues and different expectations of childbirth; she squashed a few myths and fears. She also taught us about postpartum depression and how to notice it and get help for this. It's not uncommon, and it's best treated early before it becomes a real and long-lasting problem, but when it's acknowledged and helped in the early stages, this makes a big difference to the outcome.

One of the most helpful things she told us about was the community resources available. It's reassuring to know what is out there and quite surprising, too.

These ante-natal classes covered many of the seven Cs.

- Concerns - anxieties were brought up – pain relief and privacy being two top topics.

- Care - the who did what and who would be present at the birth.

- Communication – she discussed family, friends, and work. Finding out about maternity leave was helpful since we could make our plans around this.

- Consider – points to consider include birth positions, the strange (to me) possibility of a water birth and where the delivery would take place, hospital or home birth, and the risk and values of each.

- Cesarean Section? This is a matter for an individual to discuss with their medical staff.

- Culture – I never thought about different expectations in different cultures.

Attending the ante-natal classes was an experience in itself, and I wish - I wish I had gone the first time around.

Best of all was my wife holding my hand and gazing up at me with those big, trusting eyes. I had shared her journey, I understood much of what she was going through – our pregnancy journey together was a journey that made us come even closer in our relationship.

To summarize

This section has been about the practical tasks that need attention. When you plan ahead, the financial aspects are much more manageable, and by taking care of this, you can take a huge weight off your partner's mind and let her get on with growing your baby.

When you support her by attending the prenatal classes with her, many of the concerns and questions you never knew you had are explained and answered. It also gives you and your partner a great talking point and helps you make a baby plan together.

Your role is crucial in the practical planning for the birth of your child. Being jointly involved brings you closer together and promotes a sense of sharing and understanding.

Helping Her Eat for Two

The term "eating for two" is a bit misleading, and it often makes women feel like they have permission to eat enough for two full-grown people. However, your partner's nutritional needs will undoubtedly increase over the next nine months, and it is partly your job to help make sure she healthily meets those needs. Healthcare professionals currently recommend that women gain between 25 and 35 pounds during a healthy pregnancy. These recommendations vary based on a woman's starting weight, so be sure she consults her doctor for a personalized recommendation.

On a side note, now is most certainly *not* the time to make any comments about your partner's weight, body size, or food choices. She is more emotionally vulnerable than she has ever been, and you may land yourself permanently in the dog house with one ill-chosen comment or "helpful" suggestion. The best thing you can do is help shop for and prepare healthy food choices, make sure she gets her prenatal vitamins, and be unconditionally loving and supportive. You can encourage her to eat well by setting a good example and laying off the unhealthy options yourself. There's nothing worse than tempting a pregnant woman with food she can't or shouldn't have.

During pregnancy, your partner is literally "making the baby" – in an assembly kind of way – so good ingredients are essential for a quality end product. This means that your unborn baby needs good food. Your partner also needs proper nutrition to help her deal with the physical, mental, and emotional changes and challenges she faces until the baby is born. The female body requires about 10 to 12 percent more energy when she is pregnant. Below are some of the basic nutritional requirements you should help her meet on a daily basis:

- **Six servings of fruits and vegetables:** An apple or tomato is a serving; so is half a cup of salad. Leafy green vegetables are particularly useful as they contain folic acid (see information below), which helps prevent congenital disabilities such as spina bifida.

- **Six servings of grains:** A cup of cooked pasta or rice, or a slice of wholegrain bread or a bread roll makes a serving. Whole grains are particularly useful because they, too, contain folic acid.

- **Three servings of dairy:** A large glass of milk, a small container of yogurt, or two slices of cheese. Low-fat or skim dairy products can help control weight gain.

- **Two servings of protein:** An egg, two slices of lean red meat, or two chicken drumsticks are one serving. Vegetarians can also get protein from nuts and seeds, legumes, and tofu.

Folic Acid and Other Vitamins

Folic acid, also called folate, is a B vitamin that is important to help prevent certain congenital disabilities. Eating folate-rich foods such as whole grains, chickpeas, and leafy green vegetables helps your partner reach the recommended daily allowance of 400 micrograms. Most pregnancy healthcare providers recommend upping your partner's folic acid by using vitamin supplements, even before she gets pregnant. Check the recommended amount of folic acid, as some women in a high-risk category need more, and follow your health provider's instructions.

Foods She Shouldn't Eat

Pregnant women shouldn't eat certain foods because of the risk of bacteria, such as listeria, to which pregnant women and unborn babies are incredibly vulnerable. So be sure you don't give her the following foods during pregnancy:

- Any cooked food that has been in the fridge for more than 12 hours
- Cold deli meats or pate.
- Ready-made salads from the deli or your grocery store's refrigerator section.
- Soft cheeses, like blue, ricotta, and blue vein.
- Sprouted seeds.
- Sushi, unless it only contains vegetables or fully cooked fish.
- Unpasteurized milk.
- Undercooked, or runny, eggs.

Ask your primary care provider, obstetrician, or midwife for a comprehensive list of foods and medications to avoid.

By the end of her pregnancy, your partner may be itching to eat a good bit of brie or sushi again, so a great way to celebrate your baby's birth may be to put together a platter of the things your partner's been missing out on for nine months. Start a "foods to remember after birth" list today!

You Should Get on the Wagon, Too

Your partner must avoid all kinds of harmful substances to help keep your baby healthy. Seeing you swigging a beer or inhaling sushi will maker her needlessly cranky and resentful, so show some solidarity and stay away from the same things she must avoid.

Activities to Avoid

While we're on the topic of things to avoid, you should know about some activities your partner should stay away from while she is pregnant. The following activities are not recommended for pregnant women:

- Exciting theme park rides, because of the acceleration the body experiences during the ride.
- Extreme sports and adventure sports, such as skydiving, bungee jumping, parachuting, and whitewater rafting.
- Traveling on a plane, although this mostly applies at the end of the pregnancy.
- Using permanent hair dye, because of the chemicals used in dyes.

You should ask your doctor for a comprehensive list of activities to avoid.

Chapter 2. Importance Of The Role Of Becoming A Dad

It is talked about less often, but the dad's role throughout pregnancy and delivery is an extremely important one. Your partner is in this with you, and this is their child too. Just because they did not get to feel any of the morning sickness or baby kicks does not mean that they aren't just as invested as you are in the whole process. This chapter will focus on what the dad's role is and how to work through certain feelings that arise or questions that come up. There is a myth that tends to circulate that a dad does not have to do much at all when a mother is pregnant, but that is not even close to the truth. Not only is the dad going to be the main support system, but he is also going to be learning and discovering just as the mother will.

The Importance

Feelings of cluelessness are normal for first-time dads. This is a brand new experience, and it should not be expected of every dad to know exactly what to do and when to do it. Just as the mother is going to be dealing with different changes, the father will also have to do the same thing. The main way to be a helpful father to an expecting mother is to just be there for her. Accompanying her to all of her doctor appointments is the first step. This will provide her with a sense of support, and you will also get to experience all of the same news and information that she will experience.

Try to do some research on your own time. The more you can learn about pregnancy and delivery is going to help your partner. Just as her own education on her pregnancy is valuable, your education is deemed just as valuable. Taking initiative is what makes you a great father from the very beginning. When it comes to picking out names, participate in the process! This is your chance to make a decision with your significant other. Think about the names that you like and make suggestions when the mother decides that she would like to talk about what you would like to name your new baby.

Doing housework is a great way to be helpful to an expecting mother. As her pregnancy progresses, she isn't going to be able to do all of the chores that she usually does. All of the bending down and walking around that can be avoided will help to put her body at ease. Communicate with her every chance you get. If she isn't feeling well, ask her directly what you can do for her that would help. A significant other that is willing to ask is a lot better than one who simply stands on the sidelines and waits for instructions.

What to Expect

In the beginning, you aren't going to notice that many changes. The expectant mother might feel sick more often than usual, but you can help by ensuring that she stays hydrated and well-nourished. Remind her to take her prenatal vitamins, and cook nutritious meals for her when she is hungry. In the first trimester, you shouldn't have to change much about your typical routine as a couple. The symptoms that she will be dealing with should be manageable, and if they aren't, you can take her to the doctor to see if there are any solutions that will make them easier to handle.

As the pregnancy progresses, the expecting mother is going to reach a point where she might stop working and stop driving. This is where you are going to have to pick up the slack. You will be the one driving her to her appointments, running errands, and going anywhere else that you need to go. Whether it is late-night runs to the supermarket for food or trips to the pharmacy to pick up medication, you can expect to be doing it all. This is the point where it will usually become more tiring for you. Again, if you are prepared for all of this, there is no reason for you to become stressed out at the thought of it.

When the birth plan is being created, you should have a say in this, too. While the expecting mother is going to have her own preferences, she will likely be asking you what you think about her choices. Be honest with her, and offer any helpful advice that you feel will make the labor and delivery easier. If a home birth or water birth is scheduled, do your best to make sure that everything is going to be in place when the time comes. Being a great father begins with being a great planner; think about every detail.

How to Help

Do not tell her what to do. No matter what you are communicating about, an expecting mother does not particularly need to be told what to do regarding her own body and how she is feeling. While you might have great ideas, you can bring these up to her, but don't be offended if she decides that something else is going to be better for her. Remember, you can't feel exactly what she is feeling. Being there for support and to bounce ideas off of is extremely helpful, but being bossy or controlling is not. You need to let her take the lead when it comes to her pregnancy.

Be there to listen to her. There will be times when she simply wants to vent or complain about her symptoms. Let her do this. While there might be nothing she can do but wait them out, at least she can have you there as a support system who will always lend a listening ear. She might ask you for advice if she is unsure of things and this will bring you even closer together as a couple. Each decision that the two of you make together is going to impact your baby. While you might not know exactly what you are doing if it is your first time, let those instincts kick in.

Take her shopping for baby items. Once the first trimester is over and people have been told that you are expecting a little bundle of joy, a lot of the fun can begin. Most couples create a baby registry at a store of their choosing. Aside from these items that will be given as gifts, there are still plenty of things that the parents will have to purchase as they prepare for the arrival of their child. Going shopping for these things really solidifies the idea that your baby is going to be there soon. Do things for the baby's nursery, as well. Being able to decorate and design the nursery together is a great bonding experience.

Identifying Feelings

As a soon-to-be-father, you are going to have so many emotions running through your mind and heart. While the mother usually gets to express herself more frequently, know that all of your emotions are also valid. You might be worried about how you are going to care for the baby because you are unfamiliar with what to do, but you also might be incredibly excited to mold a young mind with your own morals, values, and traditions. No matter what the case is, express yourself! The expecting mother will appreciate that she isn't alone with any of her feelings. Fathers can often take a back seat to the point where it might seem like they don't have any strong emotions, but that isn't always true.

You are about to take on several new responsibilities, all in a short matter of time. Just as the mother might have some things to change about her lifestyle when she finds out she is pregnant, so will the father. For example, if you enjoy going out on the weekends with your friends, you might need to spend more time at home as the expecting mother experiences more intense symptoms. While you cannot tell what it is like to physically feel these things, you can definitely support her as she goes through them. If any feelings come up that are overwhelming (either positive or negative), talk to her about them. She will appreciate your openness. You don't need to pretend that you know exactly what is going to happen because let's face it, you both probably don't. Pregnancy is a learning experience that you will work through together.

Sex during Pregnancy

The only reason to avoid sex during pregnancy is if either of you is not in the mood to have it. There is nothing that you will do to hurt the baby while you are having sex; that is just a myth. Feel free to be intimate with one another, and know that your baby is still going to be growing and developing just fine. If you do want to take some extra precautions, know that your partner's breasts are likely going to be more tender than usual. Any grabbing or squeezing might feel more intense than usual, so keep that in mind. Of course, if she expresses that there is any pain, you should stop immediately. Otherwise, feel free to have as much sex as you both want to, intercourse included.

A lot of couples find that the pregnancy hormones actually do a lot for the woman's arousal. She might feel extra willing and able to have sex in the beginning. As her belly begins to grow, you might have to find some new positions that allow you both to be comfortable because anything that involves her bending forward or being on her stomach for too long will understandably be uncomfortable. Much like the sleeping position, if she can lie down on her left side while you position yourself behind her, much like spooning, this tends to be a very comfortable and pleasurable position for couples who are expecting.

Consider that she might be more emotional than usual. Do your best to incorporate a lot of foreplay before you begin having sex. If you are too rough, this can be off-putting to a woman who is currently producing high amounts of hormones that make her feel more tender and loving than usual. Allow her to be the center of attention, and ask her what feels good.

Communication does not have to be a mood-killer; it will actually help you become better lovers.

Overcoming Intimacy Issues

Even though she is in the mood, you might have trouble getting into the mood yourself. This is okay, and this is normal. Pregnancy changes a lot. It forces you to think a lot more responsibly and practically than you would have before. There is also the issue of you feeling that you are going to hurt the expecting mother if you advance in any type of intimate way. Rest assured that she will be able to tell you if something hurts or if it is uncomfortable. A lot of pregnant women regularly have and enjoy sex throughout their pregnancy with no problems, physically or emotionally.

Understandably, there might still be a few things that you are worried that you will have to work through. Talk to her about your feelings. Working together, you can overcome any worries that you might have in order to get back to the core of your intimacy. Starting with simple touching and massage, these acts of intimacy can go a long way and allow you to start having sex again. She is going to appreciate all of the little things you do for her, even if they are not sexual. Opening doors for her and cooking her meals are little and intimate ways to show her that you care.

A Dad's Role during Delivery

Early Labor

As the woman enters early labor, your main job is to be her distraction. She is going to be feeling contractions, and these are uncomfortable. Do your best to take her mind off of them, but do not make her feel ignored. If she needs to complain, be her ear to listen. Read to her, talk about some of your favorite things, bring up funny memories, and do anything you can to get her mind focused on something else. If she stays too focused on the pain, her active labor is going to feel even worse. Try to get her up and moving. Walking around can alleviate a lot more pain than simply staying still. Walk her up and down the hallways if she feels like she can.

Active Labor

As you know from any classes you have taken or any research you have done, active labor means more active contractions. They are going to become stronger and closer together, and at this point, you will likely need to provide your hand for her to squeeze. Rub her back and reassure her that she is doing a great job. If you notice that she is starting to panic, try your best to get her back to a calm state of mind. Just as you learned in class, you are going to be her support system during this time. Try to work on breathing techniques that you have learned. Know that she is naturally going to be agitated and moody during this point. Allow her to have this moment because you don't know what she's feeling. She might be snappy, but know that she is definitely appreciating the little things you are doing for her.

Delivery

The moment has come - the baby is on its way! This part happens very quickly sometimes, and it can be hard to absorb everything that is going on. The most important thing that you can do here is to remain calm. If you are calm, then she is going to know that things are okay. The instant you lose your cool, she is going to feel panicked. If she is delivering vaginally, you can hold her hand and motivate her as she pushes. Encourage her to keep going and that it is almost over. In a C-section, she isn't going to be able to feel and see as much, so you can be her eyes. If she wants to know what is going on, you can describe it to her.

A Dad's Role after Delivery

There are normally two impulses that you will feel after your baby is born - you will want to cry and you will want to take photos. Both are completely valid reactions, as a miracle has just occurred. Be mindful that the mother has gone through so much to get to this point, and while she is definitely going to appreciate having pictures of the moment, she might not want a camera in her face for too long. Take a few shots, and then put the camera down so you can meet your baby together. If your baby is considered at-risk, then the baby will likely be taken to the nursery shortly after delivery so the mother can rest and the baby can be monitored. You can alternate between visiting with your child and keeping the mother company. If the baby is not at risk, the mother will be handed her child directly after giving birth.

In between all of this, you can make phone calls to inform your loved ones that the baby has finally arrived. It is going to be a surreal and joyous moment that you will never forget. When you go back to visit your partner, let her know how well the baby is doing, and also be sure to mention how amazing she was at delivering your little bundle of joy. She might still be in shock from the entire process, but keeping her calm and reassured is what will bring her back down to a calm state of being.

Some mothers who have to deviate from their birth plan might feel a little upset at this point, and if this has happened in your case, remind her that it was what needed to be done to have a healthy baby. If you tell her how great the baby is doing and that all of the right decisions were made, she will eventually get over not having the exact birth plan of her choosing. It can naturally be a very overwhelming time, and at the moment, it might feel like the doctors were making all of the decisions. Reassure her that you were there every step of the way and that you agreed with all of the decisions that were made. It will help her to know that you were looking out for her body and for your baby. From this moment on, the mother should feel your love. Make it a point that you are going to love her in every single moment, from childbirth to simply being together at home. Loving her always is how you are going to keep your own personal bond as strong as new parents.

Chapter 3. Home Preparations

Few things change the way you live as much as welcoming a baby into your life. Having a baby is like having a house guest who never cleans up after himself, cries a lot, and has more needs than you and your partner put together. Adding a baby to the family is not as simple as clearing out the spare room for him to sleep in. He needs stuff: clothes, bedding, diapers, all sorts of things you need to think about that become part of your daily life as a father.

As you count down to your baby's birth, you need to get things done to avoid hassles down the line – get those bags packed and ready for the hospital, get the bassinet and a car seat sorted out, and be prepared to go at a moment's notice. When he arrives, the chances are that you won't have a lot of time for decorating the baby's room or shopping for socks, so it's best to get those things out of the way now.

In decades past, preparing for the baby was thought of as primarily the woman's domain. The future mother alone was responsible for doing all the shopping and decorating the baby's room. However, this responsibility is split between partners more and more, and you will find that your partner, who is becoming more fatigued and weighed down by your growing bundle of joy each day, will be eternally grateful for any contributions you make to the preparation process.

In this chapter, you'll discover the ins and outs of what to look for when buying things like nursery furniture, strollers, diapers, clothes, and toys. You'll find out what a diaper rash is, how to prevent it, and how to help your baby when he's teething. You'll get checklists for everything you need to do before the birth and what you need to take with you to the hospital or have prepared for a home birth.

The point of all this information is so you can share as equally as possible in the process of getting ready for your precious little one. Your partner has taken the lion's share of the work by growing your child inside her body, so it's time for you to step up, roll up your sleeves, and get excited about shopping for baby stuff!

Getting the Right Gear

Who would have thought a baby would need so much stuff? Getting set up for a new person in your house takes a bit of thought – and a mountain of cash if you're not careful. Rather than telling you to go out and buy every bit of gear, the baby shops say you absolutely must have; this guide will tell you what you need.

First, to keep costs down, send the word around among your coworkers and friends that you're having a baby. They may have cribs, bassinets, car seats, and strollers they're no longer using. You can completely outfit a nursery for very little or even for free if you have generous friends and relatives.

The Overwhelming World of Baby Clothes

Baby clothes come in more shapes and styles than you would have thought possible. Babies don't dress like miniature adults. They hate itchy materials, fussy buttons, and other things you might put up with to be fashionable. However, because adults and not babies buy clothes, you'll find a whole spectrum of cute stuff specifically designed to appeal to adults, covered with duckies and little toy cars.

Types of Baby Clothes

Be forewarned – it's hard to resist this stuff, especially for moms-to-be. But check out what works for you before you break the bank.

- **Bodysuits** are long- or short-sleeved T-shirts that also cover the baby's diaper area and snap at the bottom for easy changing. They are handy for keeping everything tucked in, so that baby's tummy doesn't get chilly, and they also keep him looking pulled together. They're great during the summer months when a short-sleeved bodysuit can be worn by itself without pants or as pajamas.

- **Footies** are all-in-one outfits that either snap or zip up the legs and front. They're like bodysuits with leg coverings and socks. Some snap up the back, which is inconvenient. Most have feet, but you can get some without feet (called "nonfooties" or "coveralls") for summer. Most also have long sleeves.

- **Sleeping bags** (also called gowns) are like footies with sleeves but no legs, just a sack covering your baby's legs and feet. The American Academy of Pediatrics recommends not using blankets in cribs for infants up to one year, so having her wear a sleeping bag will help her stay warm. Gowns that have elastic around the bottom are also fabulous for late-night diaper changes because if her legs are bare under the sack, you can get to the diaper more easily and disturb her less.

Listing the Clothes Your Baby Needs

The following list is a guide for things you should have ready to go for your newborn baby. You can customize your list as you figure out which items work well for you. You can also tweak the list to suit the seasons. In general, baby clothes should be loose-fitting, made with breathable and soft fabric, not too tight at the neck, and easy to open and close. Keep in mind that you can go through three to four outfits a day because of diaper leaks and baby spit-up. Here's a general idea of what you need:

- **Plenty of bodysuits:** You'll need at least six, probably more.

- **Four footies:** As with bodysuits, the more, the better. These are favorite baby shower gifts.

- **Four pairs of pants of some sort:** Overalls are cute, but make sure they have snaps in the legs, so you don't have to take the whole thing off to change a diaper. Elastic waists on pants are far easier than fumbling around with zippers and snaps.

- **Four sleeping bags:** Look for cotton material instead of polar fleece or microfleece, since these fabrics are less breathable and may lead to overheating.

- **Two jackets:** Look for jackets that are easy to zip or snap, since buttons take too long to do up.

- **Two sweaters or wraparound jerseys:** Choose the kinds that don't need to go over her head. Most babies hate having things pulled over their head.

- **Plenty of pairs of socks:** Make them all the same if possible – one is always getting lost.

- **Four hats:** These should be made of a Lycra-cotton mix, so they stretch, or soft wool if they're handmade. Some babies dislike hats and try to pull them off, so look for something that snaps or ties under the chin if necessary.

- **Plenty of bibs with snaps or Velcro:** Bibs with ties can be difficult to put on. Velcro stops sticking after some washings. Some large bibs go on over baby's head.

- **Two pairs of soft shoes:** Typically, shoes that have elastic around the heel stay on better than other slip-ons. Babies don't need real shoes until they're walking outside.

- **Two pairs of gloves or mittens:** It's best to get some that clip to your baby's outerwear because these are lost easily!

Tips for Selecting Baby Clothes

Here are some tips for selecting clothes, based on the experiences of real babies and parents. Your partner will be thoroughly impressed and relieved at your knowledge of these little insights:

- Avoid anything that doesn't have a few snaps at the shoulder or an envelope-style neckband, to make pulling the clothing over her face painless.

- Avoid anything that has a back opening. Your baby will inevitably spend a lot of time laying on her back in early months, and it can't be comfortable to have snaps under you. They're also tricky to get on when you're getting her dressed.

- Avoid anything that looks like it's going to be a pain to put on. Some babies hate the process of getting dressed, and trying to tie silly ribbons when she's having a meltdown isn't anyone's idea of a good time.

- If your baby arrives in the winter, look for clothes that have folds sewn into the ends of the sleeves. These are mittens. They're also great for keeping your baby from scratching himself with those sharp newborn nails.

- If in doubt about sizing, buy clothes that are too big. At least you know junior will grow into them. Avoid the newborn or 0-3 month sizes, unless your baby is tiny or a preemie.

- If you've been given a lot of hand-me-down clothing, be aware that the fire retardant in some clothing may be worn and will not be as effective as it is in new clothes.

- You will be given a ton of new clothing as presents, so if you find you have too much, don't be afraid to take it back to the store and exchange it for something you can use in the future, like the next size up.

- Dark colors show baby spit-up much more than light colors, but light colors show baby poop much more! Just go with the colors you like.

- Handling a baby in the first few months can feel a bit tricky because she can appear fragile. Think about what steps you need to go through to put on an item of clothing. If it seems too complicated to close or open an item, don't buy it.

- When trying to determine what size your baby needs, try to go by the weight chart provided by the manufacturer. The months listed as sizes usually have very little to do with your baby's age.

Filling the Toy Box

When your baby is born, all he does for a while is poop, pee, eat, cry, sleep, and gaze at things with an unfocused stare. So, he won't need electronic gear, a racing car set, or a mini piano just yet. What he needs are things that give him a real sense of the world he's just come into – simple objects that provide new sights, shapes textures, smells, sounds, and sensations.

You can quickly provide all these characteristics just by spending time with your baby, singing to him, and touching his skin and fingers with textures like an old comb, fabric, your hair, leaves, the cat's fur, etc. As he begins to grasp and bring his hands together, things like a rattle or a chain of plastic rings can keep him fascinated for a long time.

When your baby starts teething, he looks for things to put in his mouth to push against his gums to relieve the discomfort. Many toys would double as teething rings, even if they weren't initially designed for this purpose.

Here are some good ideas for baby toys:

- **Cloth or hard cardboard books:** Look for ones with flaps or things to touch sewn into them so your baby can experience different textures. Reading to your child every day is one of the most important gifts you can give him.

- **Plastic keys:** For some reason, babies love your car keys, so give them their own set! These are great for teething too. However, nearly every baby will still prefer your keys to his, so keep yours out of his reach.

- **Play gyms:** These are mats with arms curved over the top where you can attach bright objects like soft toys or musical objects for your baby to look at as he lies on the mat. Just make sure he can't pull down anything that he shouldn't be chewing on. Nothing is safe from his gummy mouth once he's got the hang of his hands.

- **Rattles:** You can buy rattles or make your own from old plastic containers filled with noisy objects. Ensure the lid is on securely and never leave your baby alone with an object that could come apart.

- **Soft toy animals:** One of these will probably become your baby's most treasured friend, and it will never be the one you favor, so only guy stuffed animals you won't mind seeing for the next six years. Avoid button eyes and other removable parts a baby could choke on.

Remember, you probably don't need a whole lot when it comes to toys, no matter what the manufacturers tell you. Nothing beats spending time playing and exploring with your baby.

Brain development is assisted by appropriate stimulation and human contact.

To make sure toys are safe for your little one, check for any parts that may become a choking hazard and toxins, such as toxic paints. Inevitably your little guy will try to put all toys (and most other things) into his mouth, so make sure they're safe to put in his mouth.

Stroller Shopping

Strollers have evolved quite a bit since you were a child. These days, many strollers will fit together with your baby's first car seat. As a result, you can transfer the whole seat into the stroller without removing him when he's a newborn.

Baby stores are often packed with different models of strollers. This item is often one of the most significant purchases you make in the parenthood game, so take your time when shopping around.

Here are some features you should search for:

- Can the car seat attach to it? Many brands make travel systems with integrates strollers and car seats.

- Does the stroller include a fitted sunshade and weather cover?
- How easy is it to move the stroller through store doors, the doors of your house, and fold it for storage?
- How easy is it to adjust the back of the seat?
- Is the stroller rugged enough to take off-road on unpaved walkways and trails?

Choosing the Right Car Seat

Using a car seat for your most precious cargo is not optional. You may have free-ranged in your parents' car when you were little and lived to tell the tale, but sadly some children haven't survived. So, make sure you always use a car seat when traveling with your baby.

As with strollers, so many models of car seats are out there that it pays to shop around. There are different sizes according to the age and weight of your child. For the first model that you purchase, you want to search specifically for an infant car seat or a convertible infant car seat. An infant car seat is specifically used for newborns up to approximately 20 pounds or more. Many infant car seats snap handily into a base that you install into the car ahead of time using seatbelts. For the utmost safety reasons, infants should be kept in rear-facing car seats until they reach the weight limit of the rear-facing seat or are at least two years old.

Feeding, Bathing, and Entertaining

You thought you were done shopping in the baby aisle? Oh no – there's much more to fill up your house with! You'll find most of these things lurking in homes where children live:

- **Baby bathtub:** You need something to wash your baby in. The kitchen sink may work just fine for a while, but he'll eventually need something a bit larger, but not as large as the regular bathtub. Changing tables that converted to infant baths used to be common, but many parents don't have the room for them. If you do have one, it'll save some wear and tear on your back. Otherwise, you'll need something to set in the big bathtub, at least until your baby can sit up by himself. A bath support is a ramp that baby can lie back on that holds her at a 45-degree angle, so her head is safely kept out of the water. There are many different styles, and you and your baby may prefer one type to another, so shop around.

- **Bouncy chair or infant seat:** Most kids have spent time in a bouncy chair or infant seat, which is a baby chair that your baby can lie in to watch you go about your day from a better angle than lying on the floor. These seats are portable and easy to clean, and she can even sit outside in one while you're gardening. Some have built-in vibrating mechanisms that calm a fussy baby, while others have activity trays that keep baby busy period these seats come with safety straps that should be used every time you put the baby in it.

- **High chair:** When your baby starts solids, you're going to need somewhere she can sit to be fed. A wide range of high chair models is available, from chairs with an ergonomic design made of wood that hasn't been treated with chemicals to chairs with more levers and straps than a space shuttle. Having a detachable tray that you can take off and clean regularly is essential, as are safety straps so you can be sure she isn't going to wriggle her way out of it and get hurt. As an alternative to a high chair, you may want to use a model that attaches to your table. Later on, you can use a little booster seat that you strap to a normal chair.

- **Swing:** No, this isn't the kind of swing you can attach to the apple tree. This kind lives inside your house and takes up about half your living room. Baby swings can be lifesavers if you have a fussy baby because the constant movement suits him, although watching it may drive you crazy.

Making Room for the Baby

When you were growing up, do you remember how important your bedroom was? It's more than a place where a child's bed is or where his clothes are stored. It's a child sanctuary, his own special space that has all the things he loves close by. Although he won't know this for a while yet, you can start creating that individual, happy space for him before he's born. But first, we cover what every nursery needs to have. Your partner will be especially appreciative of all your efforts to help get the nursery ready. Although she may have the final say in the décor and how the furniture is arranged, you can help by making sure you have everything you need and by putting everything together for her. By doing all the heavy lifting and other manual labor, you're letting her rest and focus on her most important task – growing your baby.

Finding Functional Furniture and Gear

Here are the essential items you should get for your baby's nursery:

- **A place to sleep:** Many parents prefer to place their children in a bassinet for the first few months of their lives. Eventually, they will sleep in a crib, where they will stay until about 2 years of age. If you decide to get a used crib, be sure to research current safety recommendations for crib bars and mattresses.

- **A changing table:** You should look for a changing table that has the option of a strap to buckle around your little one when he starts rolling and twisting. The best changing table pads have washable covers and waterproof liners. It's also best to find a changing table that has drawers, so you can easily reach any essential supplies while changing the diaper.

- **A dresser or closet (or both);** Although infant clothes are tiny, they end up taking up a lot of room! Since you'll want to have multiple sizes on hand for rapid growth, you will probably fill up a small infant dresser or standard-sized closet quickly. It may benefit both you and your partner to come up with an organizational system for storing clothes of different sizes, especially if you are given a lot of hand-me-down clothes.

- **Other basic essentials:**

- A diaper pail with a pedal for hands-free opening.

- A rocking chair or glider where either parent can feed the baby. As the baby grows, you can read pre-bedtime stories and share cuddles in this chair, too.

- A bookshelf or toy box.

- Toiletries like diaper cream, wipes, and powder.

- All recommended health items, like nail clippers, a thermometer, children's liquid acetaminophen, and a snot sucker.

Decorating the Nursery

Decorating your baby's room is another way to clean out your wallet in a hurry, as there are thousands of things to put in a little person's room to add personality and style. Expectant moms have been known to get carried away so you may have to display a bit of good old male shopping rationale. Babies spend a lot of time gazing into space when they're really small, as if they're tuning into a radio show you can't hear, and like looking at high-contrast objects around them, such as black and white shapes. Keep the decorating simple. As your baby develops his taste and his needs change, transforming the nursery into a little child's room won't take a complete overhaul.

Here are some tips for keeping the decorations simple:

- Keep the colors and designs neutral, so that the room can easily be redecorated as your baby grows.

- Use pictures of close friends and family on the wall so your baby can grow up knowing who the important people are.

- Mobiles hanging from the ceiling don't have to be fancy. A string of shells hanging from driftwood can entertain a small baby, but make sure anything you hang is extremely durable, so it doesn't fall apart on the baby's head. Also, make sure the mobile is well out of a baby's reach because small pieces or hanging strings can be a choking or strangling hazard; remove the mobile when he's able to get to it.

- Use removable decals on the walls so they can be easily taken off as baby grows up and out of the nursery themes. Choose things that won't damage the wallpaper or paint.

There is infinite information out there about physical preparation for a child in your home, so don't let yourself get overwhelmed. Take the advice and information that seem practical and helpful and ignore the rest. You'll eventually learn through trial and error exactly what you need for your unique family and child.

Chapter 4. What A New Dad Needs To Know

Your Emotional Well-being in a Post-Pregnancy World

In much of the fatherhood literature out there, you will hardly find a mention of the feelings that new dads go through. These authors, well-meaning as they are, focus solely on the nitty-gritty of taking care of the baby. They forget that dads need caring for as well, or they won't be able to take care of the baby. I mean, how do you deal with the uncertainty, the isolation, and the jealousy? You will feel rotten for missing—or even wishing for—the good old days when you and your partner had just each other.

In the worst-case scenario, you will also have difficulty bonding with your child for the first few months. Engrossed with motherhood, your partner will most likely be too preoccupied with the baby to notice any of what you will be going through. In this chapter, we will examine the common emotions you can expect to feel after the baby's birth as well as the relationship changes likely to occur as a result of your bundle of joy's coming into your life.

Emotions You Can Expect to Feel

Like motherhood, fatherhood is a rollercoaster of emotions that only those who have been through it can appreciate. The most challenging thing about parenthood is the expectations that people feel to act in particular ways. You feel the pressure very deeply when everyone around you just expects you to feel happy and excited all the time. This is especially the case when people judge you for having feelings different from others in a similar position. So, you lock your real feelings deep down and put on a brave face. But how effective is that? I suggest that you take a different approach. Recognize all these emotions early on, figure out what your heart is trying to tell you, and use this to improve yourself as a father.

Excitement—but Also Helplessness

Fatherhood is exciting. It gives you an opportunity to become a full family. You have probably developed a pretty comprehensive idea of the kind of dad you would like to be already, and it is time to realize your dream. How exciting is that? At the same time, what if you fail? What if you end up being a terrible father and giving your daughter/son serious daddy issues? What if you become the reason your child struggles to form relationships later on in life?

This helplessness works very much like a curtain falling in front of all the excitement you are feeling about fatherhood and blocking all the joy off. The truth is, you cannot control how the future of your newborn child plays out. You cannot protect him/her from the falls, the heartbreaks, and other adversities s/he will encounter along the way. Before you accept this fact, you will struggle with the helplessness of your situation. Loving your child so much yet knowing that there is little you can do to protect them from the world around them will be hard.

To alleviate your feelings of helplessness, you can start by helping around the house and doing everything you can to become the caring dad for your son/daughter. Only by fostering a strong bond with your baby will you get the opportunity to be super dad and protect your child from any threats around them.

Joy—but Also Guilt

Any moments you spend bonding with your baby or supporting your partner as she handles the complicated baby care operations, like learning to breastfeed, will bring you a lot of joy. If you are bottle-feeding the baby, you will also experience the joy of feeding the baby in a huge way. It is tempting for new parents to get trapped in the baby vortex and only feel good when caring for him/her. This is especially the case when there are some challenges in the process. Knowing that you are doing everything you can to make life easier for your family just feels right.

Until you feel neglected and decide to indulge yourself a little. For example, you may decide to catch a quick game or go out for a jog to clear your head. You know, the things that bring you joy and make you appreciate life. The truth is that if you are a jogger or if you enjoy football, it forms a part of your identity. It gives you the emotional and physical energy you need to care for your baby. But the indulgence will cost you a measure of guilt. In fact, any personal time you take as a new parent comes with a lot of guilt.

Any time you feel guilty for indulging in personal pleasures, just remember that you are only as good a father as the person you are. And if you are grouchy and high-strung because you don't get to indulge in your personal pleasures anymore, you will only grow to resent the baby. I am not saying don't make sacrifices—you will definitely need to make a few. However, I would not advise giving up anything that contributes to your overall well-being.

An Outpouring of Childhood Emotions

You would think that bringing a child into the world is an opportunity for the parent to look into the future, but studies indicate that most parents experience a more backwards turn. According to attachment theoreticians, we see parenting as an opportunity to relive our own childhood—our way. For people with childhood traumas or repressed emotions from the earliest phase of their lives, parenthood can be very unsettling. If you have not had an opportunity to come to terms with your childhood, then you are in the twilight period of your innocence. In a few months, you will be welcoming your baby into the world—and coming face to face with your own childhood.

It is very important that you come to terms with your childhood emotions and create harmony in that area of your life. Because whether you like it or not, your childhood does play a part in the kind of parent you would like to be. This is even more important if you faced some traumas as a child or as a teenager.

But even if your childhood was innocent and carefree, there are some very nuanced influences that might affect your ability to parent. For example;

- If you were treated harshly after getting upset, you may have internalized that distress is an emergency which would send you into fight or flight mode. The problem with this is that your child will become the enemy any time his/her actions upset you.

- Children can be very perceptive about respect (or lack thereof) in their interactions with adults. If your parents did not treat you with due respect, you might unwittingly transfer this over to your child.

- Critical parents often raise perfectionist children, who grow up into perfectionist adults. Perfectionist adults become perfectionist parents who criticize their children and impose very high, often unachievable standards. On the flip side, perfectionist parents make their children feel like they need to *earn* their love, which can be very unsettling.

Here is the rather unsettling thing about childhood issues—they come out no matter how well your parents raised you. Unless you put in the work of figuring out your emotions, you will remain unaware of those triggers that might affect your ability to parent well. Now is the time to get ahead of these triggers and ensure that you are at peace with your childhood, before it is too late.

A Deeper Connection to Your Partner—but Also Emotional Distance

For some couples, welcoming a baby into the relationship strengthens the bond between you and makes you closer than ever before. There are times when everything just falls into place, you feel even closer to your partner, and life looks bright. This, of course, is the perfect-case scenario. The reality is often a lot less cheery.

Babies have a way of grabbing the spotlight and never letting go. From the moment she arrives, the baby will demand most (if not all) of your and your partner's attention. With the constant crying, late nights, and disrupted sleep patterns, it is very likely that you and your partner will grow somewhat distant immediately after the birth.

Paternal Postpartum Depression

In some cases, the joy of fatherhood is quickly replaced by unrelenting fear and anxiety, which soon blossoms into full-blown depression. This is called Paternal Postpartum Depression (PPPD), not to be confused with maternal postpartum depression, although there have been extensive studies showing a sizable correlation. Men with partners going through maternal postpartum depression are as much as 50% more susceptible to getting PPPD. If getting depression following your daughter's/son's birth sounds tragic, that is because it is. Fathers going through PPPD tend to fixate on problems, blow them out of proportion, and may even lash out.

The last thing anyone in your household needs is to be dealing with a full-grown man throwing tantrums or drinking right now. You know you are supposed to be the protector and the provider, but how are you supposed to handle *this* particular issue? DO NOT let the old-school notions of the invincible man twist your thinking. Failing to get help is the assured way of harming your family. You need to get help.

You should visit a therapist if you are exhibiting the following signs:

- You quarrel and get angry with others a lot more frequently.
- You are using alcohol and street drugs as a coping mechanism to deal with your stress.
- You are irritable and frustrated, especially when there is no apparent cause for your irritability.
- You feel pent-up and exhibit signs of violent behavior.
- You gain a significant amount of weight or you lose a good amount of it.
- You feel increasingly isolated from your friends and family, especially your wife and child.
- You get stressed easily and have trouble shaking off the stress once it takes root.

- You engage in impulsive behaviors and take unnecessary risks, such as having an affair or driving dangerously.
- You have the feeling that nothing will ever be good again. You are discouraged.
- You experience constant headaches, indigestion, and body aches.
- You are unmotivated and have trouble concentrating on any given task.
- You lose interest in things that previously gave you pleasure such as sex, your hobbies, or work.
- You use work as a shield between you and the world and between you and your family.
- Even while you spend all your time at the office (work), you are not as productive as you should be.
- You feel that you are not the kind of man you would like to be. You are disappointed in yourself.
- You are entertaining thoughts about death and suicide.

Postpartum depression may develop as a result of a difficult adjustment to having a baby in your life. In the event that you are part of the 50% of men who get PPPD along with their partners, you are in an even more precarious situation. You need to get help as soon as possible to ensure the continued safety of your child.

Why It Happens

Essentially, PPPD is happening because the role of fatherhood is changing. The expectations that men and society have about male parenting have experienced a seismic shift in the last few decades. We are now asking of ourselves things that our ancestors would never have dreamed of. The fear and anxiety that causes PPPD indicates the lack of preparedness that men have for their changing fatherhood roles. If you are taking turns waking up to comfort the baby in the middle of the night, the lack of sufficient sleep increases your chances of anxiety.

Then there are the additional pressures that men feel, such as the financial stress of caring for a new member of the family, balancing work (and your old life) with caregiving, and lower levels of testosterone. All these factors play a part in opening men up to emotional and mental discord much like it does with mothers.

How to Deal With It

Dealing with PPPD requires a comprehensive approach entailing:

Overcoming the stigma

You probably feel the need to be strong and capable a lot more strongly now that you are a father, which is why you will find it rather difficult to own up to your postpartum depression. But here's the thing—you are not the only one! Men suffer from depressive mood disorders all the time; it is just that they don't go announcing it. And if you really want to become strong, then be strong for your family. Admit that you need help to harness your fears and anxieties and channel them productively, and go get that help!

Seeking professional help

The good thing about treatments for PPPD is that they tend to be short and effective. For example, cognitive behavior therapy gives you the tools you need to understand how your emotions affect your behavior. It takes an average of three months to complete. Other therapies like relationship management improve self-worth and give you the tools you need to build the quality of your relationships. In general, therapy gives you power and makes you feel more in control of your own thoughts and feelings.

Reaching out

Sometimes you develop depressive symptoms because you get too much into your own head. You start judging yourself (harshly, of course) and you fall short of your own expectations. You can get a better perspective on your merit as a father by talking to other fathers and sharing your frustrations and your fears. Talk to people who are already dads—your own father, a co-worker, a stranger at the park—and get their perspectives. You might be surprised to find that you have always been a pretty good dad. And if nothing else, this will take some of the pressure off.

P.S.

I cannot reiterate this enough: caring for your family starts with caring for yourself. Self-care is the ultimate remedy to postpartum depression. And this goes for you and your partner as well. It is no good (especially for the baby) if you give up your pleasure pursuits only to have your well-being take a dip.

Your Relationship After Baby's Arrival

Relationships tend to change as soon as the baby arrives, and usually not for the better. Some couples accept less intimacy as part of becoming new parents, but this is not how it is meant to be. And even though your relationship will definitely change after the birth of a child, you can do something about it. In this section, we will touch on some common relationship issues and ways that you can handle them.

Common Relationship Issues

As soon as the baby arrives, you discover that there are too many things that need to be done. Even worse, there will always be something to do at any given time. This limits your freedom to indulge both as a person and as a couple.

In some cases, fathers have to fight to get their partners to accept their views on how to take care of the baby. It is a no-win situation whereby you feel like a jerk if you contradict your wife. After all, she did carry the baby for nine months and suffer the pains of breastfeeding, etc. When you don't voice your views, you become resentful and the relationship suffers.

As a couple, you are either sleeping late and waking up early or sleeping early and waking up super early or multiple times in the night. One or both of you will be suffering from sleep deprivation, making you snappy and reactive—not exactly the recipe for a happy couple.

Like it or not, sex plays a huge part in fostering intimacy between any romantic couple. But with the crazy hours and never-ending baby care, you will hardly ever have time for it. Moreover, your partner will probably be feeling very unsexy in light of her recent bodily changes. It also can take weeks for a mother's body to heal after childbirth, which can make the experience of sex highly unpleasurable.

A relationship will only be as good as the people in it are feeling. At some point, the personal frustrations will come pouring out and sour everything. So, if you are not getting any "me" time, your entire relationship is very likely to suffer as well.

The extended family can be a huge blessing when they take over the duties of caring for the baby and giving you and your partner the chance to get some alone time, apart and together. At the same time, constantly having family around will make it harder to hit the levels of intimacy you are used to.

How to Handle These Problems

You can solve any relationship issues that crop up by simply talking about it in a calm and rational manner. It is better to have a fight about a contentious issue and get it out of the way than to have it bubble under the surface and poison your relationship in the shadows.

As her companion, your job is to look out for your partner. You should always keep in mind that your partner was affected by the birth and the immense changes in her body more than you. If you recognize the signs of postpartum depression, support her as she seeks help and be there for her along the way as well.

With a baby between you, you cannot just take a break from the relationship "to think things over." However, you can definitely take a timeout when things get too heated and unproductive. You can use the Lily and Marshall "pause" button from "How I Met Your Mother" to avoid escalating issues and to gain some perspective.

Your partner shutting down and going into "mommy" mode all the time will probably be the biggest hindrance you face as you try to revive the relationship flame. Sometimes all you need is to show her that you are in this together. You can do this by engaging in parenting tasks together. As you bond over the baby, you will find that it gets easier to talk her into scheduling 20 to 30 minutes per day for just the two of you to reconnect.

How to Strengthen Your Relationship After the Baby

Overcoming the issues that come up along the way is not nearly enough if you are in a loving, caring relationship. You need to find ways of using the baby to make you and your partner a stronger couple. After all, the stronger you are, the better you will be as parents.

Understand that you are a team

Most couples make the mistake of making baby care a competition or a game of one-upping each other. The small misgivings that competition brings add up, and not in anyone's favor.

Laugh together

The importance of laughter in a relationship cannot be overlooked. If you can laugh together, then you can love together. And if you can love together, nothing can get between you.

Embrace the predictability

The worst mistake you can make as a new parent is to keep clinging to the old ways when you made decisions on the fly. Accept the fact that, to a large extent, spontaneity will disappear from your life instead of trying to "live in the moment" and other such bachelor nonsense. Plan ahead for bonding moments and anything you want to do with your family.

Practice patience

Among the things that you will need to be patient about is your partner's infatuation with the baby. For the first couple of days, she will probably spend all her waking time in service to the baby. As the weeks roll by, she will keep cutting down until you can have your fair share of both her and the baby. Keep in mind that nothing is permanent and your situation (whatever it might be) will improve substantially in a few months.

Play your part

Baby care responsibilities are to be shared with your partner. In the first few days/weeks, your partner will probably take on every aspect of baby care. This is not an opening for you to abdicate. At some point, you will have to come in and handle a few things. The more the duties you are able to help out with, the better off you will both be as a team.

Chapter 5. The Attention Of Dads For The First Time

The way to work on fostering a strong bond with your child is by engaging in bonding activities. Instead of moaning that your paternal bond is not as strong as you would like it to be, take a more proactive route and throw yourself at the challenge of falling in love with the baby. In this section, I will highlight eighteen surefire activities to bring you and baby together.

Cuddle Your Baby as Often as Possible

As much as you need to work up your affection towards the baby, you also need to stir that affection in him/her towards you. Babies are usually very attached to their mothers, a result of nine months of close contact followed by breastfeeding and ceaseless doting. Your opportunity to start establishing a connection starts after birth. Get in as much cradling as you can, including holding the baby in the breastfeeding position as you feed him/her. This gives you ample chances to establish eye contact and a deeper connection. Throw in kisses and smooches as well for full measure.

Heavens know that baby's soft skin feels heavenly on your lips.

Get in as Much Skin Contact as Possible

Mothers bond with the baby through skin contact starting from birth and proceeding onwards. You can also nurture your bond with the baby by seeking to establish contact through kisses, bathing, and playtime. Babies enjoy the freedom of being naked, and in a warm enough room, you can play with him/her in a diaper without worrying about giving her a cold. It does help that a baby in diapers looks super cute as well!

Become Baby's Comforter of Second Resort

In the deep of night, when your partner is too tired to wake up to comfort the baby, you will win yourself some important points by becoming the rescuer. You can even have your partner set you up by delaying her response (especially when you are teaching the baby to self-soothe) so that you can come in and save the moment. Your face and your arms should be the next best thing after mommy's face and arms to the baby. Yeah, do not even think about knocking her from the throne. It is impossible.

Make the Baby Laugh

You know that thing about the fun dad—it is well worth a shot. You can take it upon yourself to catalogue all the things that the baby enjoys (those that make her laugh) and those that she doesn't much care for, the ones that elicit nothing above a blank stare. If you are the parent with whom the baby has most fun, you will feel more valuable to the baby and enjoy your time together so much more.

Unlock Your Inner Child With the Baby

You will probably never get a better opportunity to indulge in your most playful tendencies than with your baby. Even though this might not be plausible in the first few months, you can indulge in silly playtime with the baby as much as you like. The better you get at showing your baby a good time, the stronger the bond between you will be even when s/he grows up. Even though your play activities will change over time, the bond will remain just as strong as ever.

Talk to the Baby

You might think that the baby does not understand what you are saying and you are absolutely right, but talking to her goes a long way in nurturing a strong bond between you two. Let your baby become accustomed to your voice. This way, she begins to associate your voice with all the fun activities that you engage in together. Nothing beats receiving an automatic smile from the baby or having him/her extend those tiny hands towards you in eagerness to spend time with you.

Sing

Whether it is jingles or lullabies, songs contain the sounds that elicit the most delightful response to a baby. Singing also makes your voice so much more attractive, making the baby more responsive. Even if she only gives you nothing more than a curious look the first few times, keep on doing it. At some point she will reward you with a smile, then a giggle, and before you know it she will be supporting herself on the bassinet and dancing along to the tune. When the baby goes to sleep to the sound of your voice, it reinforces the bond even further.

Read the Baby a Bedtime Story

The time before sleep is very suitable for strengthening parental bonds with the baby. Read a bedtime story, even if your baby doesn't understand. They'll be soothed by your voice. As your baby develops an attachment to these stories, s/he will also develop an affection for your voice, and in extension, to you.

Watch Your Baby Sleeping

Singing your baby to sleep allows you to establish a stronger bond in him, but watching as he sleeps reinforces the strength of your attachment to the baby. Just imagining how marvelous it is that you formed a full person—mixed in with the cuteness of a sleeping baby—will make you feel more emotional about the baby than you have ever felt before.

Wear the Baby

If you have any negative notions about carrying your baby in a sling, you need to throw them away and get a special sling just for you. More than a stroller, a sling helps you to establish contact with the baby, which is very important in fostering a stronger bond. A sling allows the baby to get used to your smell, your movements, and your touch. It also reinforces the sense of security and safety.

Take Pictures and Family Videos!

Sometimes all you need to do is gaze at the baby through the camera to feel the stirrings of affection. Starting from the hospital bed, you should designate yourself the official cameraman of your small family. Take birth videos, birthday videos, play date videos, record all the firsts, and basically take it upon yourself to document your baby's entire childhood. S/he will be glad to have something with which to relate to those parts of the early life where memories blur as we age. Not to mention the fact that you will have an endless repository of film and pictures to remind yourself of those special moments for you and your partner.

Fill your Role With Grace

When it comes down to it, your baby will probably prefer your partner over you for pretty much all the activities you enjoy doing with him/her. Do not take it personally when the baby cries, fusses, or prefers your partner as a soother. You have a lot of ground to cover to catch up with your partner and you will probably not catch up for years yet. This is not the time for jealousy. The important thing is that your baby is well tended to; sometimes you just have to accept that you are not the man for the job.

Bath Time Bonding

Babies love playing around with water. As soon as she can, your baby will be splashing and giggling so much during bath time you will probably even forget about the cleaning part. All the fun you have during baths will translate into valuable bonding time for the both of you. As I suggested before, there is great value in carving out bath time as a baby-and-me time.

Dance Together

As soon as the baby can move, you can start dancing together to her favorite music. Even before s/he can move, you can just move around with her/him and trust in the magic of music to do the rest for you.

Try a Baby Massage

There is ample evidence on the benefits of massage in fostering muscle development, soothing tummy aches, and inducing relaxation leading to better sleep in babies. You can take it upon yourself to be your baby's masseuse. A massage provides you with ample opportunities to strengthen the bond with the baby, starting with the skin contact, the simple pleasure of a well-done massage, and the relaxation it gives the baby. Just be careful to apply the lightest touches possible so as not to harm your baby's delicate bone structure. Also use massage oils to reduce the chances of giving the baby friction burns and chafing.

Love on Your Partner in Front of the Baby

Babies can be surprisingly possessive of the people they love. This is why firstborn children have so much trouble accepting the arrival of new siblings. Your baby's first love will be your partner and s/he might be very possessive. In her own little world, mommy's kisses are for her alone. Engaging in some PDA in front of her and then plastering her with smooches is a great way to reinforce the notion of mutual love amongst the three of you.

Take Part in Bedtime Routines

You can decide to partake in any bedtime activities with your partner, but you definitely should never miss out. In fact, bedtime is a great time to reinforce the image of the three of you as a family by loving on each other.

Practice Patience

Patience will become even more of a virtue to you when you are having trouble connecting with your baby. Most of these suggestions take time to bear fruit, and you will probably get a lot of frustrations along the way. However, if you keep at it and never give up, you will one day look and realize that you have long established a deep connection with your baby boy or baby girl. It also helps to think about all these activities in less transactional terms. Sing your baby a lullaby because s/he needs one to soothe them to sleep, not to get a smile or love. Wear the baby because you want to help out, not to get something out of it. Think of it this way—would you be doing any of these things if you had fallen in love with the baby at first sight right from the hospital? You would most probably be doing a lot of these things anyways.

Chapter 6. How To Be An Excellent Parent And Partner

Caring for Baby and Helping Your Partner

Every baby is different, and every family is different. In the coming days, weeks, and months, you'll discover how to read and care for your child like no one else ever will – except for Mom, that is. Now is the time to put into practice all the training you received for caring for your baby. Much of it will be trial and error. Don't worry; there is no such thing as a perfect parent. Everyone has made plenty of silly parenting mistakes, especially in the early days, and their children have survived and thrived despite these errors.

The most vital thing you can do is help your partner as much as possible. She is going to be exhausted and hormonal from the experience of the birth for several days or even weeks, especially if she had a cesarean delivery. As a result, you'll still need to do the lion's share of household work without complaint. It will take quite a bit of time before she is able to be up and about to her pre-pregnancy abilities.

If you are bottle feeding, you can share equally in feeding your baby, especially at night. Taking turns with feeding is one of the best ways to help the two of you cope with the unbelievable strain of sleep deprivation you'll experience in the first several weeks of parenthood. If your partner is breastfeeding, you can still help tremendously by changing the diaper and making sure baby is clean and dressed before handing him off to mom for a feeding.

Other ways in which you can help are making sure mom and baby get to scheduled check-ups, cooking meals, and making sure any well-meaning guests don't overstay their welcome. Everyone will be eager to meet your new little one, but your priority should be making sure your partner does not get overwhelmed, and the baby is not disturbed or overstressed by too many guests. Try to space out visitors, so you don't see more than one or two people each day, and set aside certain days in which you receive no visitors, so your new family can bond and relax together.

Baby Blues or Something More Serious?

About day three after birth, mom may start feeling a bit low. This is perfectly normal and should pass. She may burst into tears for no reason that she can explain or just feel overwhelmed by responsibility. If she had a hard pregnancy and is looking forward to getting her body back, finding it isn't "back" yet may be very disappointing. Chances are she will also be sore in all sorts of places. Performing simple personal hygiene tasks or even just going to the toilet can be really tricky and uncomfortable. On top of all that is the fact that her hormone levels have gone through yet another dramatic shift, which significantly affects her mood and body. Do your dad thing and try to support your partner by helping out, telling her she's amazing and enjoying your baby.

These initial baby blues have nothing to do with postpartum depression, which is likely to come later if your partner ends up experiencing it. Feeling "the blues" is one thing, being in a black hole is another. That's how some people describe postpartum depression (PPD). The condition is associated with mothers for the most part, with an estimated 10 to 15 percent of mothers suffering from PPD. What's less well-known is that three to ten percent of fathers can suffer from PPD, too. This is a serious condition that cannot be ignored without significant consequences.

Recognize the Signs of PPD

Knowing about and recognizing some of the signs of PPD can assist you to seek help for yourself or your partner if either of you experience PPD. Symptoms to look for include the following:

- Anxiety or panic attacks.
- Feelings of hopelessness.
- Frequent crying spells.
- Loss of energy or appetite.
- Loss of enjoyment in everyday activities or your baby.
- Loss of sex drive.
- Mood swings.
- The trouble with sleeping even when the baby is settled.

- Prolonged feelings of sadness, with nothing to look forward to.
- Suicidal thoughts.

Every case is different. If you feel you or your partner may have PPD, talk to each other about how you're feeling and see your doctor.

Getting Help

If your partner has PPD, supporting her may seem like an impossible task, but you can help in lots of ways. Try some of these ideas:

- Arrange a time for you to spend together, just the two of you. Regular "us" time can help destress both of you and share some common ground again.
- Let her talk while you listen, or involve a friend she feels comfortable talking to.
- Take over more of the housework and baby care so she can try to get some sleep. If you can't take on everything, enlist the support of family and friends.

- Treat her to a special gift, a date night, or some pampering at a spa.

- Make sure she is following up with any therapies, doctor appointments, or medications needed.

For additional PPD support and help for either one of you, try some of the following ideas:

- Talk to your doctor. He can offer a wide range of options like counseling or medications. He may also know of local sources for support groups.

- Find support in your community — many hospitals host groups dealing with PPD. Online groups can also be a lifesaver.

- Get some exercise. Feeling fit and active can lift your mood or the mood of your partner. Around 30 minutes of daily activity is all that is needed to release mood-enhancing hormones.

- Talk to family and friends. You might be amazed at how anxious people are to help, and many of them may have had similar experiences.

Postpartum depression is temporary, and you can find a way to help yourself or your partner through it. If you feel lost, take stock and get some help.

Keep Communicating!

Make sure you and your partner communicate well, no matter how stressful things get. Touch bases frequently to be sure you are on the same page regarding feeding the baby, changing diapers, and beginning to establish a routine. Find out how she's feeling about returning to work, if that was her plan, and be supportive if she needs to voice her unsteady emotions. More than anything else, keeping the communication lines open will help you and your partner remain close and work as a team as you navigate the unknown waters of new parenthood together.

How to Support the New Mom: The First Day Home

There are many useful ways a partner can help the new mom. These are some of those ideas:

1. Screen the visitors if necessary.
2. Keep her company.

3. Do as much cleaning and cooking as possible or organize other people to do the additional chores.

4. Provide some communication: With everything on mom's mind, it might just take a good talk to clear the air and make her day. You cannot rely on your mind reading skills. Ask what she needs.

These are all excellent tips especially when Mom and baby arrive home. The first few days will be hectic setting new patterns. Life will seem upside down for a while.

Dad's Share Breastfeeding Time

It is a known fact, dads cannot share with the breastfeeding process, but that leaves many other tasks that can be accomplished by the proud parent. Dad can still get the baby up and change the diaper. A nursing pillow and a glass of water would be an added convenience for mom. If all it takes is a bottle, (Dad) you can warm that up for Mom and baby.

Support Partner's Parenting Decisions

Support makes the job of mom and dad a simpler process when both parties can make informed decisions. Letting mom know that she is doing a great job can be all it takes to turn a blue mood into a happy event.

Be sure you (Dad) ask if it is okay you are taking over on some of the tasks. Your partner might believe she has to do all of the work. Even though she needs the help, sometimes, it is difficult to admit it.

More Feel-Good Things Dad Can Do For Mom

- **Meal Planning**: Take over some or all of the meal planning and cooking. You can begin with a healthy breakfast as a surprise to get her day off to the right start to be sure she is eating three nutritious meals every day. She has probably been too busy with the baby to realize it was her mealtime which can often happen with young children, especially newborns.

- **A Massage**: After giving birth, mom could probably use a nice massage. After holding the baby in her arms all day, it could be a welcomed release. You—Dad—

could offer her a pleasant massage. Remember, though; Mom might not be inclined to reciprocate. You know the rules of giving and not receiving; she will let you know when it is adult playtime.

- **Appreciate Her**: Let her know she is appreciated and buy her a personal present for no reason—just because you care. Give Mom the credit card and send her out to buy a few new clothes. Neither the clothes worn before pregnancy—nor the maternity clothes fit. New moms never have any clothes which can leave her feeling miserable without any nice, comfy clothes to wear.

- **It is Okay:** Tell her that it is okay the home is a bit messier than usual; provide your services for a cleanup routine. Moms are usually too distracted to realize the mounting load of laundry or the sink full of baby bottles. Cleaning just isn't on the top of the 'to-do' list.

- **Encouragement**: Always provide encouragement and let her know you are proud of her and the way she is handling her new motherhood job. Frequently, let her know how much you love her, and provide praise for her great job.

- **Make Mom Happy:** Suggest an outing (all on her own or with a friend) for a haircut/color so she can feel a bit more glamorous. Run her a bath and purchase some 'girly' magazines (something that isn't related to her new baby). Let her take over control of the remotes.

Things Dads Do With the Baby

It is more to making Mom happy than just on the first few days home. It takes 100% of her time, but Dad can take many of the chores away. These are just a few of those fun events:

- Go for a walk with the baby so Mom can have some quiet time.
- Take the middle of the night feeding. The 2 a.m. bottle sometimes comes quickly to an over-tired mom.
- Take the early morning feeding so mom can sleep in

for the day. If she is using breast milk; you can always have an extra bottle ready in the fridge.

- Cuddle with the crying baby if he/she won't stop crying; mom is flustered.

- If other children are in the home; take some of the responsibility from Mom's hands. You (Dad) can take the carpool or manage the dentist appoint for one day.

Make sure Dad knows how to change the dirty diapers and perform bath duties. Many new mothers find it enjoyable and helpful when specific jobs are set aside for Dad. It gives Mom a time to look forward to if it has been a stressful day.

Additional Tips for Dad

The first month of your baby's life is also going to be the most challenging. You've already been through so much hype with the baby shower, the packing, the hospital, and the birth, now your baby is here, then what? Postpartum depression is not just for moms it happens to dads to, at a rate of about 10% to be exact.

The month that follows your child's birth will need all the strength and patience you can muster as it is a time of adjustment for your baby and for you. Get through this and the rest should be a breeze. Well, a breeze compared to the first month at least.

1. Change your idea of 'normal' – That life you had before baby was born if officially gone the second he comes out. What 'normal' you were used to is out the window and needs to be replaced with a life that has baby included in all things.

You may think 'I can still have a nice dinner out with the wife, just hire a baby sitter'. Your baby will be in your thoughts for at least a small part of that night, if not all night. And even if he might not be at all, he still might be in your wife's mind which still affects your date.

We aren't trying to turn you off to life with kids here, we are stating the facts so you, as a new dad or dad to be will know exactly what to expect.

2. Sleep deprivation – this comes with the package and not just for mom but for you too. As previously mentioned, babies feed at least 8 times a day, that's every 3 hours and when mom wakes up at 2 in the morning, you could very easily say to yourself 'well I don't breast feed so what use am i?' be there for support, or change a diaper.

Both parents will be sleep deprived somehow, and every opportunity you see for a nap, you may want to take. It would be nice if you let your partner nap first as though you both nay be tired, she has been breast feeding which consumes a lot of energy, she is also recovering from child birth, especially if she has had a C-section which may take weeks to heal.

3. Keep an eye on mom – having the baby blues after baby is born is completely normal but there is a thin line between that and post-partum depression. If you suspect her of having this legitimate medical disorder, it will need treatment and you should contact your physician for

advice immediately and urge her to share her feelings with you.

4. How do you feel? – make sure you ask yourself this and acknowledge your feelings. This could be one of two things: you either feel left out because mom is doing everything to, with, and for baby and you feel useless; or you may feel overwhelmed by the amount of things that you need to do. Remember that your emotional state matters a lot, it is up to you to take care of mom and baby's well-being and you need to be the strongest for them both.

It is ok to take a break every now and then by meeting up with some friends either out or at home, just make sure you aren't out for too long or that your friends don't overstay their welcome.

5. Pamper mom – before baby came, there was already a bulk of chores to be done, washing dishes and clothes, sweeping and vacuuming, cooking, etc. now that baby is here that chore load more than doubled. Offer to do

some of it for her so she can take a break. Double the cuddle dosage.

6. Fair parenting – this means that the duties are split equally between mommy and daddy. Much too often, mom does the bulk of what needs to be done for baby. Yu need to take on some of this responsibility yourself and show mom that you can do it right. Don't make excuses such as 'oh but you do it better' no one knows all this baby stuff upfront, your wife is learning just as you are.

Example: there was a new dad friend of mine that got assigned (by mom) to wash the baby bottles. Mom walks into the kitchen and notices him washing them out without using the bottle brush or any soap for the matter to which dad responds 'its water based cleaning' what happened next was nothing short of world war 3.

7. Confidence – learn as you go and be confident about it, odds are you are just being paranoid. Know that your wife and baby need you now and will always need you.

111

Chapter 7. The Step By Step Guide From The Temperature Of The Bottle To The Bond With Your New Baby

Bringing a baby home isn't like bringing home a new PlayStation or a new LED TV. You don't get an instruction manual that comes with the box, and you're pretty much left to figure things out on your own. If you're not careful, you might be completely shocked by how much your life is going to change once a baby actually comes into the mix. This is especially true if you're the kind of person who likes to live life by a strict routine. All of those routines will get thrown out the window when you have a newborn at home. Even when it starts to feel like you've got some sort of new system going on that works well for you and your partner, a baby is more than capable of finding a way to mess up your system. There's so much power that can come from such a small package.

While all of this may seem like troubling news to you, there's really not much reason to worry. Very few parents ever really know what they're doing when it comes to raising their kids because it's always a case-to-case thing. What works for one set of parents might not necessarily work for all, and that's fine. You just have to try to find what works for you, your partner, and your child. Eventually, the three of you will figure things out and really get the hang of parenting. It might take a while, but that's okay. This chapter will help orient you on the many things you may need to know about finally bringing a baby home from the hospital.

How to Hold the Baby the Right Way

Unfortunately, holding a baby the right way isn't necessarily going to come as naturally to some parents. That's fine. A lot of parents make the mistake of overthinking the process, believing that a baby is this infinitely delicate creature that can break at the slightest touch. There are also some parents who aren't familiar with the weak and sensitive points of a baby's anatomy, and so they end up manhandling a baby like it's a slice of meat from the butcher shop. If you're either one of those parents, then read up.

The first thing that you need to do is wash your hands. A baby's immune system is strong, but it isn't as strong as it should be. This is why you need to keep the baby in as sterile and clean an environment as possible. Cleanse your hands with soap and water or hand sanitizer before holding your baby.

Next, make yourself comfortable. It's not just about finding a position that's comfortable for your baby to be in. You also want to make sure that you're comfortable with holding that position for a prolonged period of time. When holding the baby, be sure to support the head and neck. They are the heaviest parts, but the baby's neck isn't yet strong enough to support the head. This is especially true for the first four months of a baby's life.

Popular Holding Positions:

- Cradle Hold. This is when you cross your arms along your body so that it forms a kind of cradle for your baby. To do this properly, make sure that the baby's head is resting gently on the crook of your elbow with the rest of its body laying across your forearm. Use your free hand to add additional support to the baby's head.

- Shoulder Hold. With the shoulder hold, the baby's body is parallel to yours with its head resting gently on your chest or shoulder. One hand should be supporting the baby's bottom as its torso lays flat against your upper body. Use your other hand to support the baby's head and neck to keep it flush against your body.

- Belly Hold. The belly hold is a lot like the cradle hold except the baby is face down. This is an ideal position for when your baby is gassy and you need to burp it.

- Lap Hold. The lap hold is a great position to place your baby in while you're seated. Place the baby on your lap with your feet planted firmly on the ground. Position their head between your knees and make sure that your hands are supporting it. The baby should be lying on top of your forearms which serve as its mattress.

How to Change the Baby

Whether you like it or not, you're going to have to learn how to properly change your baby's diaper. It's a rather sticky situation (pun intended), but it's part of the duties of being a new dad. It's definitely going to seem a little challenging at first, but you'll eventually get the hang of it with more practice. Before you can get started, make sure that you prepare everything that you need for the task:

- fresh diapers
- diaper cream or ointment
- changing pad or table
- trash bin or bag
- fresh clothes (if necessary)

While baby wipes are generally marketed as safe for babies, you have to know that your newborn's skin is rather sensitive. This means that they are more prone to rashes and irritation. If that's the case with your baby, ditch the wipes and clean your baby's butt with good old warm water and soap. However, if you find a pair of wipes that don't irritate your baby's skin, you are free to use those as well.

The first thing you need to do when changing a baby's diaper is to wash your hands. Then, gather all of your supplies and make sure you have everything within arm's reach. Lay your baby down on a stable changing pad or table. Unfasten their diaper tabs by gently raising their bottoms off the surface of the pad. Grasp their ankles and slowly lift their legs upward as you slide the diaper off them. Clean the baby with a wet cloth or wipes. Dispose of the used diaper and wipes into a trash bag when done. Slide a clean diaper under your baby and apply the creams or ointments before fastening it close. Clean and disinfect the changing pad before stowing it away after use.

Bonding with the Baby

When the baby is born, it automatically gets the chance to bond with its mother through skin-to-skin contact. It's a standard medical protocol, but there's also something that's deeply primal and natural about the bond between a mother and her child. However, that doesn't mean that dads shouldn't get to bond with their kids too. In fact, you should definitely be working hard at establishing that connection with your baby. Here are some ways that you can go about doing so:

Skin-to-Skin Contact

There are many scientific biological benefits to skin-to-skin contact, and this shouldn't only be reserved for the child's mother. As the dad, you should also be coming into contact with your child so as to establish that connection with them. Another way that you can build your intimacy with your baby is by looking at it straight in its eyes. Their consciousness may not be fully developed yet, but their senses certainly are.

Sing to Your Baby

You don't have to be Frank Sinatra or anything. But the point of singing to your baby is essentially allowing them to orient themselves to the sound of your voice. Again, their consciousness might not be fully formed yet, but they can hear you. And if they associate the sound of your voice to environments of comfort, then that will further build on the bond between the two of you. If you're not totally comfortable with singing to your child for whatever reason, you can also try to just read to them. They might not understand what you're saying, but it still serves the same effect as singing to your child.

Bathe Your Baby

Newborns don't typically require frequent bathing. But when you get the chance, offer to get into the tub with your newborn. Again, a bath is typically a very relaxing experience for a baby. It's crucial that they are able to associate these relaxing experiences and feelings with your presence. This will allow them to feel more comfortable and at ease whenever they are with you.

Wear Your Baby

Babywearing simply means wearing your baby on you in a carrier or sling. It's a great way for you and your child to really bond with one another. There's something very comforting in the way the child is suspended close to your chest, and they really do enjoy that feeling. Aside from that, wearing your child is incredibly practical for when you need to run errands or perform certain chores that require your hands. You still get to bond with your child while being productive in other aspects of your life.

Swaddling 101

Sometimes, nurses or midwives will teach you and your partner how to swaddle your baby after they are born. Swaddling is a great way to comfort your baby because it somewhat simulates the sensation of being inside a mother's womb. It's essentially just the act of wrapping a baby into a blanket like a burrito. We've already talked about how a baby isn't really capable of regulating its own internal temperature so soon after birth. Swaddling will help keep them warm as they develop that natural skill and response. Wrapping the baby snuggly in a blanket will also prevent them from flailing their limbs out and about, which could potentially startle the baby and interrupt their sleep.

To swaddle your baby correctly, remember to:

1. Lay the swaddling blanket out flat onto a soft surface with one corner of the blanket folded down.

2. Lay the baby face-up in the middle of the blanket with its head directly underneath the folded corner.

3. Straighten the baby's right arm and wrap the right corner of the blanket across her body so that the ends are now tucked in between her left arm.

4. Repeat the process with the other side of the blanket.

5. Twist or fold the bottom of the blanket and tuck it under one side of the baby. You want to twist or fold it tight enough so that it's snug without being constrictive.

6. You can test the tightness of the swaddle by checking if the baby has enough room to move its hips around.

The Struggle of Feeding

When it comes to feeding your child, you might be feeling completely helpless and useless due to the fact that you can't necessarily offer them your nipple. But just because you can't produce milk yourself doesn't mean that you can't help to feed your baby. You can still make yourself useful by:

- bringing the baby to your partner when it's time to feed

- helping position the baby so that it's easier for them to latch

- preparing nursing pads, lanolin cream, tissues, water, or anything else your partner might need to make her more comfortable

- putting the baby back to sleep after feeding

- feeding the baby with bottled formula

Depending on the decision that you and your partner make with regards to the baby's feeding, you might already choose to start using a bottle. If that's the case, then you can play an even bigger role as a dad in the feeding process because you can contribute by handling the feeding yourself.

Now, as to whether you should breastfeed your baby for a certain period or not is entirely up to you. There are arguments on both sides. One camp says that doing only breastfeeding allows for more natural nutrients from the mother's milk and that it's healthier for the baby. It also helps strengthen the bond between a mother and child even further. But then there are also those who say that not all babies or mothers take to breastfeeding too well, and so the baby ends up becoming deprived of valuable nutrients.

Regardless, it's best for you to make that decision together, but always place more weight on what your partner thinks. After all, it's her body that serves as the subject of your discussion. With that out of the way, let's assume that you've both decided to start bottle-feeding the baby. Here's how you can do it right:

1. Wash your hands before you do anything.

2. Next, you need to prepare the milk. Sometimes, you can get the milk directly from your partner's breast via a dedicated breast pump. If not, you can also make use of formula that you can buy in a store. Either way, you should prepare that milk beforehand by warming it up. You don't want to heat the milk up too hot and fast. Heating it up too much could potentially remove some of the valuable nutrients that a baby needs. If you've frozen breastmilk in the freezer, allow it to thaw overnight before warming it up.

3. Make sure that the bottle and all its parts are clean and sanitized before placing the milk inside. When the milk is in the bottle, mix everything thoroughly to prevent any lumps. Formula only stays good for two hours

from preparation or for 24 hours in the refrigerator.

4. Warm the bottle using a stove, faucet, or dedicated bottle warmer. If you use a stove, place a small pot with water on top of the stove on low heat. Allow the lukewarm water to warm the contents of the bottle by placing it in the middle of the pot. You can also just choose to run the bottle under warm water through your faucet.

5. There are two positions by which you can hold the baby for feeding. The first one is to cradle the baby like we discussed earlier on how to properly hold your child. Use your free hand to help support the bottle as your baby latches onto it. The second is to have the baby in a seated upright position as you gradually hold the bottle to the baby's mouth. Either way is fine. It's just a matter of finding a position that's most comfortable for you and the baby.

6. If your baby is having a hard time with latching, feel free to experiment with

different bottles and different latches. Sometimes, it can just really take the right latch that your baby can grow accustomed to.

7. Lastly, you need to burp your baby after feeding. You can do this by gently placing the baby over your shoulder with one hand completely supporting its bottom. The other hand should be gently tapping its back to allow for the baby to expel any buildup of gases inside its body.

Co-Sleeping

Co-sleeping has gotten a bad rap in the parenting community. There are many who will say that co-sleeping puts the baby in an unnecessarily risky position when sharing a bed with their parents. Most commonly, the possibility of sudden infant death syndrome (SIDS) is what a lot of parents fear when sharing a bed with a baby. Personally, I would not recommend co-sleeping for parents but I also believe that parents should be able to make their own decisions based on the information that is presented to them. That's why I think it's best to give both sides of the argument on this matter.

On the other side of the aisle, there are parents who say that co-sleeping is good because it promotes bonding and connection between the parent and child. Another added benefit of co-sleeping is that it makes middle-of-the-night nursing a lot easier for moms. If you and your partner are considering co-sleeping, it might be best to weigh out the pros and cons to help you come to a more informed decision.

Pros

1. Parents and babies get more sleep. Usually, babies wake up in the middle of the night needing to nurse. In a co-sleeping setup, the mom could begin the nursing process before the baby wakes up fully, allowing everyone to go back to sleep easier. It also relieves parents of the duty of having to wake up, get up, walk over to where the baby is, and nurse them back to sleep.

2. It lessens the likelihood of nighttime separation anxiety for both the parents and the baby.

3. It makes parents feel more bonded and connected to their babies.

4. Babies feel more secure and safe as they sleep.

Cons

1. Babies may develop an unnecessary sleep dependence or crutch with their parents.

2. Your sleeping times may not be in sync.

3. You don't get alone time with your partner anymore (which is important to some parents).

4. There is an increased risk of SIDS or suffocation.

Again, there really is no wrong or right answer here as there are pros and cons for either option. But if you do decide to share your bed with a baby, make sure that you consult your doctor on how you can best go about doing so. It may also help to consult other parents who have tried both options so that you can get their first-hand perspectives.

Crib vs. Bassinet

When your baby comes, should you get a bassinet or a crib? Is there even really any difference? Well, apparently, there is. According to the Consumer Product Safety Commission (CPSC), a bassinet is a "small bed designed primarily to provide sleeping accommodations for infants that is supported by freestanding legs, a stationary frame/stand, a wheeled base or a rocking base, or that can swing relative to a stationary base."

On the other hand, the CPSC defines a standard crib as a baby bed designed to provide sleeping accommodations with interior dimensions of 28 inches in width x 52 inches in length. It should have a flame-resistant mattress and no mesh, nets, or screens as a material in the build of its frame. There are numerous other crib standards that aim to prevent the risk of deaths and injuries from falls or entrapment.

When it comes to which one is better for you, unfortunately, there is no definitive answer. Like it is with many other aspects of parenting, it all depends on your own preferences and personal parenting philosophy. A bassinet might seem like a more alluring choice at first. However, most bassinets aren't made to hold occupants that weigh more than 15 to 20 pounds. This means that a crib might be the more logical and economical choice, especially for long-term use.

Another factor to take into consideration is size. Bassinets tend to be smaller and are better suited for a small living space. Also, smaller babies tend to like the semi-cramped feeling of being in a bassinet. As far as build quality and construction goes, there are well-made examples of each option, and it really just depends on how they are manufactured at that point. Again, there is no definitive answer here, so it's up to you and your partner to decide which option would be best for your family.

Sleeping Parents

When you bring a newborn home, you can expect sleep to be a scarce commodity. You aren't going to get much of it. That's just the sad reality of being a new parent. But that's okay. If other parents were able to get through it, then you should be able to as well. To help with your sleep deprivation, always try to remember the following tips:

> 1. Sleep whenever you can. When the opportunity arises for you to catch

some sleep, grab it. You would be surprised at how refreshing even just a 15- or 20-minute nap can be for someone who is practically running on fumes.

2. Take turns. Your partner might have to be up a lot because she's the one who has to feed the baby if you're doing just pure breastfeeding. So, whenever the time calls for anything other than breastfeeding, she should be the one getting sleep, and you should be the one who's awake. It's all about teamwork.

3. Establish a routine. As hard as it might be, if you are able to establish even just a semblance of a routine, that can really help you in firming up your sleep cycles as parents.

4. Don't forget to exercise. It can be very easy to forget about your own physical health when you're obsessing over the baby. But having a good exercise routine can actually help you fall asleep easier when you have the time.

5. Slow down on the caffeine. It can really mess up your body's natural sleeping rhythm. If necessary, have some fruit instead as a way to wake yourself up.

Sleep is absolutely precious. Don't take it for granted. There's no way you would be as effective a parent if you lacked sleep.

Bathing the Baby

Bathing your baby can be one of the best ways to really build that bond and connection between parent and child. However, you've got to remind yourself that a baby is fairly delicate, and you can't bathe a baby the same way that you would bathe yourself.

1. The first thing that you want to do when it's time to bathe your baby is to make sure that you have all your supplies ready. You can't leave your baby in the bath to fetch a missing item just because you forgot it somewhere else.

2. Next, you've got to make sure that the water is nice and warm. Babies aren't able to regulate their body

temperatures well. It's up to you to make sure that they don't get too cold while in the bath.

3. As you slide your baby into the bath, make sure that you have a good grip. Gently slide your baby into the bath feet first with one hand supporting its bottom and the other arm cradling its head.

4. Gently lather just a little bit of soap all around the baby's body. They won't need a lot of it. Make sure that you are using only a mild soap for this.

5. Start with the baby's face and work your way down to its toes. Make sure that you rub as gently as possible. Make use of a soft clean cloth to really dig into some of the baby's nooks and crannies.

6. Use a tear-free shampoo to cleanse the baby's hair. Lather the shampoo and gently massage the baby's scalp.

7. Rinse the baby off and dry by gently patting its entire body with a soft towel. Make sure that you don't rub

the baby's skin, even though the towel is made of soft fabric. Tapping will do the trick.

Don't Forget about the Pictures!

Yes, of course, it's always important to live in the present and be mindful in the moments that unfold as you get to know your baby. But that doesn't mean that you can't take pictures either. When both you and your child grow older, you are going to want to have these snapshots as a device to help you look back on these novel times that you share together as a young family. It's nice to preserve these moments in your head as precious memories, but it would also be nice to have them stored in your phone or computer too.

Chapter 8. Plan And Refine Your Childcare Style

From the onset, you need to determine the kind of parents you will be as a team. Sometimes having a different parenting style from your partner can help your children as they seek guidance in the future, but it also creates room for strife if one parent is permissive and the other is authoritative. At the same time, you do not want to become the father whose style of parenting is "do what your mother says." This all boils down to the kind of adult you want to make of your baby. Attachment styles are formed in infancy. For example, teaching a baby to self-soothe teaches him/her to be independent—a lesson that sticks even later on in life.

As a man, you should avoid becoming too dependent on your mom, sister or other extended family members in determining your parenting style. You can use your own childhood as an inspiration, but the decision you make should be mutually agreeable to both of you.

Ask For Guidance

Ultimately, there is someone out there who has a better idea about parenting than you do. Whether it is a member of your family with high-performing children or a parenting expert, there is no problem with asking for help. The important thing is to make sure that you take the decision with your partner as a cohesive unit.

Get Help

Help comes in many styles and forms, including books on parenting that are available on the internet. There is absolutely no shame in admitting that you need help. In fact, this admission could be the one thing that saves you from making a huge mistake.

Choose A (Authoritative) Parenting Style And Stick To It

There are four parenting styles, namely authoritarian, authoritative, permissive, and uninvolved. Authoritarian parents combine demands for total obedience with low responsiveness to a child's needs while authoritative ones combine high expectations with sufficient support to create a supportive and nurturing environment for the child to grow.

On the other hand, permissive parents place very little demands on their children while offering massive support. Finally, uninvolved parents provide neither structure nor support for the child.

Studies indicate that authoritative parenting is the most effective way of raising a child. It facilitates proper growth and maturity in a child academically, socially, emotionally, and personality-wise.

Defend Your Personality Style

Regardless of the studies, there will be people who will question the way you decide to parent your baby. It is important to learn how to defend yourself against these attacks. Or you might decide to disregard the criticism and simply ignore the attacks. Ultimately, it is completely up to you and your partner to decide how you want to raise your child. No one but you has the right to decide (and enforce) your style of parenting.

Types of Dad

What type of dad are you? Dads will also have a complex on their ideas on how to raise kids and their definition of what it might take to be a good father. Somewhat different to the ideals of women and moms, these dad types might give you an idea of what you might be like as a father based on your present personality. Remember, there is no need to directly categorize yourself with any item listed below or with any bits of information from several categories. The best father is the one who is honest with himself and his inhibitions.

1. The head of the household – the man that lives in the traditional sense of being the head of the household. If you belong in this category then you have the very good intention of doing whatever it takes to provide your family with everything they want and need.

As a father or father to be in this category you may be working not just for the anticipation of your new child or for the present but also for plans well into the future where you feel the need to open up accounts for a college fund and such.

A father that provides for his family is sure to gain all the respect he deserves through the provision of comfort and need but remember that too much work and no play makes daddy very dull. Remember who and what you are working towards instead of keeping your mind focused fully on work. Children will love you for the time you spend with them more than what you are able to give them.

Get on the floor and play with your child, never forget that they need a father to grow up with and your presence should be seen and felt as much as possible.

Through placing yourself in the head of the household position you set an example to your child, no matter how young they are, about the sheer importance of responsibility. Children who grow up with these fathers develop and early sense of purpose and set goals for themselves in order to later on achieve the bigger picture.

> 2. The cool dad – this often applies to younger fathers or fathers that have kids during the beginning of their professional life where reputation is just being formed, or alternatively, during the peak of their professional achievements.

We've all seen kids like this; the ones that sue the latest Bugaboo for a week, then switch over to their Maclaren for the park, or maybe a Quinny for going around shopping. Don't know what we're talking about, new dads? The cool dad would; these are high end and very expensive strollers. Or maybe the kid with the Ralph Lauren diaper bag, you know, that one wearing the pink Burberry plaid jumper?

The cool dad will be concerned with other things as well, of course, but one of his top priorities is that his child learns at an early age that you need to dress to impress and get your way in the world.

Children with these types of dads grow up with only the best of the best because nothing else will do. These dads have good intentions of feeling the need to provide their child with the best, as parents we all have this compulsion, but dads in this category make it one of their top priorities

> 3. Overprotective – the Mary Poppins of Dads. You'll know if you're in this category as you would have probably finished all the pregnancy books before your wife even has. Your child hasn't been born yet but you already put their name down for that prep pre-

school that needs a 3 year in advance reservation.

This type of dad is the kind that goes out not just with a stroller but with baby reigns, a carrier, sunblock, insect repellant, a full first aid kit, maybe even a helmet. They have it all planned out from when the child wakes up to the healthiest and most beneficial breakfast, morning activities, lunch, nap, etc.

Remember to give mom a say in how your child is raised and that even if sticking to a routine and schedule is important, a little spontaneity never hurt anyone. If your kid wants to go into that newly opened bookstore that you just saw a block back, go there even if it isn't on the schedule.

Kids can't be tied down to a strict military style regimen, this will only frustrate them. Make sure the schedule is kept with slightly blurred borders and leeway for any activity that might just pop up. Let the kids be kids and let them make their own mistakes.

Children who grow up with overprotective fathers often will reach a point where they test the limits and hence learn to defend themselves.

These children will become strong and turn into the ones that fight for what they believe is right.

> 4. Clueless – ALL dads are clueless when they just start out so don't worry. We'll call this category the foundation to which your 'daddy-ness' is built. Before going into daddy training with mom or through reading all those maternity books, you might not have a clue how things are done.

Dads in this category can't tell the difference between the front and back of a diaper. This category has dads that are blank canvases just waiting to be painted on. If you feel that you are absolutely clueless or that you could benefit from a little extra knowledge, seek it out. Never be ashamed to ask questions if the outcome offers you the possibility of being better prepared for your child's arrival.

Some clueless fathers may end up as the playmate dad and make mom feel as though she has an extra 'big kid' instead of a husband. This is NOT A BAD THING. Playmate dads are great, they are the ones that form close bonds with their kids, they are there at every soccer game, they are the ones jumping into swimming pools and playing catch together, and they watch cartoons and play video games.

Children who grow up with this kind of dad develop a very close relationship with them and through this close relationship, children are more likely to let out what they feel and everything they may be going through, this gives you the opportunity as a father to guide them through their trials better.

Conclusion

Regardless of the kind of situation through which you are becoming a father, you should start preparing for this eventuality long before conception. To strengthen the bond between you and the baby, become as involved as you possibly can in the growth and development process of the baby during pregnancy. This means attending doctor's appointments, going with your partner to birthing classes, and working on the more physically demanding preparations like baby-proofing the house and working on the nursery.

Through the course of the pregnancy, your partner will go through different phases of physical and emotional changes. You can expect to go through massive changes to the relationship, including how you engage in sexual activity. You will either have a partner with a stronger sex drive throughout the pregnancy, one whose sexual drive decreases as the pregnancy advances, one with a reduced one throughout, or one that fluctuates as the months go by. You should make sure that you flow with the tide and avoid making your partner feel pressured either way.

However much you try, you will never understand how it feels to have a baby growing inside you. That is why the man's job during pregnancy is always to support his partner in whatever she is going through. Worry about things like the nursery and baby-proofing the house so that she does not have to do it.

In preparation for the baby's birth, it is important that you have a serious discussion with your partner as to the kind of birth you are going to have. Natural birth is recommended for any woman who can pull it off because it gives the best recovery time for the woman and has some very useful benefits for the child. To settle on the best one, sit down for an honest, professionally guided talk with your doctor well in advance of the birth. You should also talk with your partner about your role in the birth. There are great benefits to participating in the birth of your baby, prominent among which is an improved ability to bond with your baby early on and lending much-needed support to your partner through this stressful time.

But whether you participate in the delivery directly or not, your role will be that of a committed assistant from the onset of labor to the arrival of your baby into the universe. Worry about things like the hospital bag so that she does not have to do it. You should also be the buffer between your partner and friends and family who come to lend their support during and after labor. You should also be your partner's advocate among the delivery staff. Ensure that the delivery goes how you and your partner envisioned it, even if others oppose.

In the early days of your baby's arrival at home, you will find yourself getting overwhelmed with chores and endless tasks. However, the most important moments will be those entailing direct care for the baby. Even though you will struggle to do it right in the first few weeks or so, you will find a lot of joy in activities like bathing, feeding, and dressing up the baby. You will probably find some of the other activities like changing the diaper and burping the baby hard to master and rather disgusting (ew, poop!), but they are just as important for establishing a connection with your baby.

Speaking of which, some fathers struggle to connect with their babies in the first few days. This is quite normal, but it does not mean that you have to accept it. You might find yourself dealing with paternal detachment, a condition that affects quite a large number of men and affects the amount of affection between daddy and baby. If you find any excuse to avoid spending time with the baby, you wish for the old stress-free days, or you envy the relationship between your partner and the baby, then chances are that you haven't formed a very strong bond with the baby yet.

You should engage in nurturing and play activities with the baby as much as possible to make sure that you build your relationship and that you fall in love with the baby. The only thing a father is supposed to feel about his daughter/son is overpowering love and protectiveness. Resentment and indifference have no place in this very special bond.

Sometimes the reason why you are not having any success bonding with your baby is because you have not dealt with the emotions their birth evokes in you. Dealing with excitement, helplessness, joy, spousal emotional distance, and an outpouring of issues from your own childhood can be rather taxing emotionally. Especially if you do not deal with your childhood emotional baggage, you will find it very difficult to bond. In these times, you will be more like a child and less like the father, which will further complicate the relationship. You have to deal with these emotions so that you can deal with any red flags holding you back from being a great parent.

Another mistake a lot of fathers make is ignoring their postpartum depression even when it continues to wreak havoc on their emotional and mental well-being. If the birth of your baby did not give you joy, or if you are feeling frustrated and exhibiting the signs of violence, you should seek help as soon as possible. However, to do this, you must first overcome the stigma. As much as you are expected to be a "man" you must now keep in mind that you are someone's father. You have to take care of your emotional well-being and throw off some of those stereotypes about manhood that you have been holding on to.

Do not be surprised if your relationship with your mate takes the backseat in the weeks and months following the baby's birth. However, do not accept this as the new normal. You must keep working on the older relationship because it directly impacts the emotional well-being of the baby.

It is inevitable that family and friends will be very interested in the birth of your child. And as your wife puts in much of the work, you will have to learn how to deal with all the family members and friends who will visit your home to wish you well. Most importantly, you will have to strike the perfect balance between letting them in and preserving the familial bonds you have established with your partner and your child. You will also have to learn how to defend your parenting style against people who disagree and those who will criticize you.

The final piece of advice I have for you is how to deal with special circumstances. The most common include dealing with infertility, single fatherhood, and gay parenting. In the first scenario, the most important thing is to find a way forward and follow through on it as a couple. Avoid blaming each other and go into whatever solution you decide to use as a couple with as much excitement as you would embrace a traditional childbearing situation. With single parenthood, the two most important things that you must do is deal with your emotions regarding the absence of the mother as well as how to utilize the help of friends and family. With gay fatherhood, make sure that you assign roles in advance and create a strong support system around your baby.

So, there you have it—the most comprehensive guide on fatherhood that you will find anywhere on the internet. As promised, I have tackled those uniquely male issues that fathers encounter in the process of procreating. There is nothing difficult about it. In fact, it can be a pretty exciting time for you, your partner, and your baby. As long as you are willing to put in the time and effort, you will easily become the perfect example of fatherhood for everyone around you. And most importantly, you will be literally the best daddy in the world for your son/daughter right at his/her birth.

Thank you for walking with me through this journey. It gives me enormous pleasure to have the opportunity to pass on all the knowledge I have accumulated over the years pertaining to baby care for daddies. I also hope that you find this book enlightening enough to warrant a favorable review. Help me get this information to first time daddies everywhere!